Are You Looking For:

- A way to avoid colds?
- A sound reducing diet?
- Help for "female trouble?"
- A really effective tonic?
- A safe source for drinking water?
- Fresh, natural foods all year around?

They're all here—along with much more remarkable, yet true, health information—gathered and presented by Linda Clark, one of today's most respected nutrition reporters as well as a bestselling author of sixteen books.

The Best of Linda Clark

Some Unusual Approaches to Health

Linda Clark, M.A.

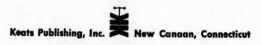
Keats Publishing, Inc. New Canaan, Connecticut

Since I am a nutritional reporter only, I have reported all available information in this book, and cannot correspond with readers nor answer questions in connection with any of the subjects included here.

Since I am not a practicing nutritionist nor a doctor, neither can I prescribe, or advise readers on their personal problems.

Linda A. Clark

THE BEST OF LINDA CLARK
Some Unusual Approaches to Health

Copyright © 1976 by Linda Clark

Parts of this book were previously published in
Let's Live and *The Total You* magazines
and are used with permission

ISBN: 87983-062-X

Library of Congress Catalog Card Number: 75-46081

Printed in the United States of America

Keats Publishing, Inc.
36 Grove Street (Box 876), New Canaan, Connecticut 06840

Contents

The Issue Is Survival

DURING A TRUCK STRIKE a while back, empty spaces began appearing on grocery and supermarket shelves as shortages developed. One of these shortages was canned cat food. A friend owned a cat named Gladstone who, like many pets, had distinct likes and dislikes and would eat only one brand and flavor of cat food. Unfortunately, his favorite brand became unavailable and Gladstone would have no other. As the truck strike stretched out from days to a week or longer, the owner brought home at least fifteen different brands of other cat food only to have Gladstone turn up his nose at them all. For one week Gladstone staged his own hunger strike, refusing all food. Finally, his anxious owner discovered a few cans of Gladstone's favorite brand after a search of smaller stores. Gladstone fell to and devoured them, his first food in over a week. Fortunately, the truck strike ended soon after.

A freight car, backing up for loading at a macaroni factory, slipped its moorings and smashed into the factory, causing $200,000 damage and closing the plant for indefinite repairs. It turned out that macaroni plants are somewhat scarce and that this one supplied 40 percent of all macaroni products in Hawaii and in all of the Southwest. Of course, macaroni shortages resulted.

A fire in a telephone exchange in New York City knocked out 150,000 telephones in one area for a couple of weeks. A small rash of fires in other exchanges followed. Business ground to a halt, for some small own-

1

ers permanently. It all proved that a working communications system is indispensable today.

What is the connection between these seemingly unrelated episodes? Shortages can appear at any moment, due to different causes. That truck strike could happen again, and be prolonged and create problems for people as well as pets. Instead of Gladstone's dilemma, the shortage of milk for a baby might result and be far more serious. And like the macaroni plant, other types of food-producing plants could be immobilized for other reasons than an errant freight car—skyrocketing prices, a strike, a shortage of raw materials or a power shortage. Or a plant could be struck by lightning, an incendiary bomb, or sabotage. Or dependable communication or transportation could be cut off. After Watergate, we now realize that anything could happen these days. And does.

But don't go away yet. There are other possibilities. All we need to do is to look back to the last few years, during which time we have witnessed gasoline shortages, shortages and rising prices of meat and other foods, rail and mail strikes in Canada, and farm workers' strikes in the United States. Near my home in California, during the height of one summer when garden produce should have been abundant and cheap, acres upon acres of lettuce and fresh vegetables were rotting on the ground for lack of pickers who were on strike. The incredible result was that the growers plowed under all of this precious food, creating shortages and raising prices of that which *was* available. And all without advance notice!

That same summer, earthquakes struck in Nicaragua, Mexico, and Colombia, leaving people without food, water and supplies. Riots in Chile closed stores and halted transportation. Power failures, especially on the East Coast of the United States during an extended heat wave, created havoc. Every year, much destruction is caused by such natural disasters as floods, droughts, hurricanes, tornadoes and late spring blizzards, as well as earthquakes. The earthquake in Guatemala is a recent example.

Top this off with shipments of United States wheat to Russia and United States beef to Japan and Canada—all producing still greater food shortages, still higher prices and mocking those who have insisted it couldn't happen here.

The money crisis is now well entrenched. In some places unemployment is climbing; inflation continues to soar.

Robert L. Preston, fiery economist, lecturer and author of the books *Wake Up America* and *How to Prepare for the Coming Crash*, is warning about the waning buying power of our money. Again, for those who believe "It can't happen here," Mr. Preston points out that it already has. For example, our dollar had already been devalued 36 percent on the world market before the floating value of currency was stabilized.

It is the speed with which such things can happen which is so incredible. Two friends took a vacation cruise to Alaska in the late summer of 1973. When they left San Francisco, conditions were relatively "normal." By the time they returned, two short weeks later, beef had practically disappeared from the market; prices in general had shot higher; consumers as well as restaurants were in a near-panic; and on another front, the Food and Drug Administration had announced that vitamins A and D in their accustomed doses were to become prescription items. The vacationers felt as if they had returned to the wrong country.

What Can We Do?

What is the solution for your protection? A survival program begun *now!* No one knows when (or if) an

3

emergency will happen, but it certainly won't hurt to be prepared.

The Bible has warned against holocausts. Religious groups, including the Mormons (members of the Church of Jesus Christ of Latter Day Saints) have long recommended storing survival supplies against emergencies. I am told the Mormons are now urging their members to take faster action. Of course, no one can accurately predict the time of occurrence of any disaster such as an earthquake, though some have tried.

Many are predicting worldwide famine and suggest a survival program which should last for two weeks. The Mormons are urging food survival units or kits for twelve, fifteen, and twenty-four months—just in case. Those who have experienced earthquakes or power failures could have already made use of survival supplies. Like taking an umbrella for a rainy day, you may not need it, but if you do, you will be glad you did. As Preston says, "It is better to be a year too soon than one day too late!"

How to Start

Before you collect your stockpile for survival, decide where you are going to store it. One family keeps theirs in a walled-off corner room of their basement. It is cool on the cement floor, and an air vent is installed on the wall, hidden from the outside by the shrubbery. Another person has only a warm attic. But with screened open windows for cross ventilation, it is better than nothing. (A fan might help on warmer days.) An apartment dweller has no place except the space beneath the bed springs, but he uses it. Another family, wondering if a basement might become inaccessible after an earthquake, stored their supplies in a woodshed, some distance away from the house. A woman, living alone, had an outdoor cupboard built against an outside wall of her small house, already too small for additional indoor storage space. A barn, a garage, a lean-to are all possibilities. Figure out the best solution for you.

What to Store?

I did not realize so much survival information was available until I began to look for it. It could fill a book. In fact, it has already filled several books. In this limited space, I can only give you hints to start your thinking and recommend some excellent books to start your reading.

Here are some lists of supplies to get you started. Keep a notebook handy and jot down other possibilities to fit your family, your needs, your circumstances, as they occur to you. You need not spend a vast sum immediately. Put in a few essentials as you can and keep adding. Also, *keep rotating foods*. Put the newer acquisitions behind the older foods. *Use those toward the front first, before they get too old or spoil.* Replace them immediately from the rear.

Don't, like one woman, fill your freezer with forty loaves of bread, excluding more nutritious food. And don't go on a carbohydrate binge because of protein shortages. Store and eat foods which keep you well, not just fill you up. Don't buy junk.

Now for those lists.

Foods

There are several categories of foods to include in your survival program:

- Fresh, grown indoors or outdoors (see Special Preparation Methods).
- Frozen, home or commercial, stored in freezer.
- Refrigerated, stored in auxiliary refrigerator(s).
- Canned, home or commercial.
- Dried. If properly dried, these foods may be the

most successful of all (see Additional Reading list and Special Preparation Methods and Special Supplies (5). Freeze-dried food can be kept at room temperature.
- Fermented foods: sauerkraut, fermented vegetables, juices. (See Additional Reading list.)

In addition to the above, store only the most highly nutritious items available. These will supply body building and repairing nutrients as well as free vitamins and minerals.

Other Suggestions

- Brewer's yeast. Keeps indefinitely and contains B vitamins, many minerals and amino acids (protein factors). This is an energy food as well as a reducing food (no carbohydrates). It serves as a quick pickup when added to juice or water.
- Your favorite protein powder to add to liquid. If you have not found one with an acceptable flavor, see Special Supplies (1).
- Desiccated liver for vitamin B-12, or other glandular tablets or powders for protein.
- Flavorings: whole sea salt (contains all minerals); blackstrap molasses (contains many minerals); fructose (see Special Supplies (1)), a newly-discovered safer product than regular sugar; honey; apple cider vinegar. (Use one teaspoon each of honey and apple cider vinegar in a glass of water for a refreshing drink, supplying minerals and natural acid to help digest protein, iron and calcium. It, too, provides a pickup.)
- Granola. Use and replace often for freshness.
- Peanut butter. A tablespoonful between meals supplies energy, allays hunger for hours.
- Natural oils. Keep in dark-colored containers in

refrigerator. Butter, margarine. Refrigerate and
replace often.
- Nuts, particularly almonds and pecans. Best
kept in the shell for protection.
- Seeds for sprouting: mung beans, alfalfa seeds,
sunflower seeds and others (see Special Preparation Methods and Special Supplies (3)).
- Beverages: herb teas and coffee substitute.
- Homemade yogurt (see Additional Reading
list).
- Kefir, also homemade. (See book in Additional
Reading list and source of starter in Special Supplies (2).)
- Powdered milk. The use of powdered skim
milk in large amounts is now being questioned,
partly because of its lack of fat, which is found
in whole milk (also in powdered form); partly
because of a high content of galactose which is
an antagonist to vitamin B-2 (riboflavin).
However, since this program is presumably not
for life, but for a short time, it may be necessary
for babies and children, and can be served on
granola, in soups, drinks, etc. Pets may accept it,
too. Spray-dried milk is preferable (most canned
fluid milks now contain additives).
- Foods for babies and pets (remember Gladstone).
- Grains (see Special Supplies (3)). Grains are
of great importance and should be stored in large
amounts, such as fifty-pound bags. Wheat can be
used for sprouting or growing mineral-rich wheat
grass (see Special Preparation Methods).
However, wheat is not the only nutritious grain.
Rye, brown rice, buckwheat, oats and millet are
excellent. These grains should be kept cool or refrigerated in airtight containers. One family

has stored wheat in tight glass containers in a cool basement for five years without insect or rodent invasion. Many people place a bay leaf here and there in the grain to discourage weevils.

Buckwheat is said to be the closest to animal protein of all plant sources, according to recent research (4). It can be served as cooked groats or ground into flour for pancakes. Buckwheat seeds can be used to produce buckwheat lettuce, high in rutin, found to strengthen capillaries (see Special Preparation Methods).

Rye has been relatively ignored. According to the late Dr. Royal Lee, animal tests have revealed that rye develops muscles, whereas wheat promotes fat formation. The Finnish athletes who eat rye instead of wheat have walked away with honors compared with wheat-eating competitors in the Olympic games. Rye eaters are usually leaner than wheat eaters and whereas many people are unknowingly allergic to wheat, they are not disturbed by rye. Rye bread, crackers or grain may be stored, but not too long. Grain keeps longer.

Oats rank next to rye as a muscle builder. The best oats are steel cut and they do not need to be cooked on the stove, merely soaked overnight in hot water in a thermos.

Brown rice, from health food stores, is incredibly delicious. It, too, can be put into a thermos for final cooking. Gena Larson's suggestion is to use 1⅓ cups of brown rice to 2½ cups of water and ½ teaspoon of sea salt and 1 teaspoon of salad oil.

Add rice to salted water in kettle, and bring to full rolling boil. Spoon into thermos bottle, previously heated with hot water, then emptied. There should be a little space at the neck of the bottle. Seal and put on the cap. Lay bottle on its side and let cook overnight, or for

6 to 8 hours. Reheat for serving if necessary. Thermos cooking of whole grains and cereal is also possible.

The keeping qualities of grains vary. Wheat is supposed to keep up to fifteen years; rye, five years; and brown rice (which can turn rancid), eighteen months. Use and store accordingly.

Supplements

Supplements are a *must*, of course. Vitamin C for detoxification, fevers and infections, together with a calcium tablet to be taken as a buffer for each 1,000 mgs of C, are imperative on a survival program.

- Alfalfa tablets not only detoxify, but supply minerals and vitamins.
- Calcium calms nerves, protects teeth, encourages sleep.
- Vitamin E aids circulation.

Add other vitamins as desired. An all-in-one supplement is also a must for survival purposes. Read labels; ask your health food store for suggestions.

Cell salts, together with the wonderful little book (see Additional Reading list) which explains which salt to use for each disturbance, are invaluable. Cell salts are minerals in easily assimilated form. The combination called "Nerve Tonic" is superb—a safe tranquilizer.

Digestants HCl and/or digestive enzymes are available from health food stores.

Water

You can live for some time without food, but you cannot live long without water. Robert Preston states that the absolute minimum of water needed is one gallon of water per person per day. Water can be stored in plastic, although glass is preferable. (The Food and Drug Administration is discouraging indefinite storage of some beverages in plastic.) Beer companies will often sell fifteen- or twenty-gallon stainless steel kegs with bottom spigots for a reasonable amount. Several of these filled with the best water you can find make a good start.

Gallon jars and five-gallon tins also make fine containers. As a matter of routine, all empty canning jars can be filled with water until needed.

Used oil drums, incidentally, are all right for holding water for uses other than drinking.

For Water Purification

1. Boil water vigorously one to three minutes. This will remove bacteria but not radioactivity. (Clorox may do that.)

2. There are several substances to use for water purification. One is in the form of tablets and available in drug stores. (Follow directions on label.) Tincture of iodine, found on most home medicine shelves, can be used to purify small amounts of water by adding and stirring well:

- 3 drops in each quart of clear water
- 6 drops in each quart of cloudy water
- 12 drops in each gallon of clear water
- 24 drops in each gallon of cloudy water

A friend who travels widely always takes with her a dropper bottle of Clorox. She adds one drop to an eight-ounce glass of water and has avoided infections picked up by others who did not purify their water.

Robert Preston suggests the following method for water purification with Clorox:

- 2 drops in 1 quart of clear water
- 4 drops in 1 quart of cloudy water
- 8 drops in 1 gallon of clear water
- 15 drops in 1 gallon of cloudy water
- ½ teaspoon in 5 gallons of clear water
- 1 teaspoon in 5 gallons of cloudy water

For purifying fruits and vegetables (not organically grown—contaminated with sprays, etc.) use the following method:

Add ½ teaspoon of Clorox to 1 gallon of water, obtained from the usual supply. Into this bath place the fruits or vegetables to soak. The thin-skinned fruits and leafy vegetables will require 10 minutes. The root vegetables and heavy-skinned fruits will require 15 to 20 minutes. *Make a fresh bath for each group.* Remove from bleach bath and place in a fresh-water bath for 10 to 15 minutes.

Special Preparation Methods

Dried Foods

Properly dried foods are perhaps the most useful of all for survival storage. They take up little space, last indefinitely, retain all natural vitamins and minerals; or if meat, fish, jerky, or pemmican, retain all protein factors (amino acids). Freeze-dried foods can be delicious.

Many commercially dried foods contain additives. You will find an excellent book on the Additional Reading list which shows you how to dry foods at home successfully, using homemade equipment or purchasing a unit, in parts or completely assembled (see Special Supplies (1)). Fruits, vegetables, meat and fish can be dried within a few hours.

The Mormons, who supply survival units or kits for various lengths of time, include dried foods only.

Do not store too many sweet dried fruits such as raisins, dates and prunes. They are high in sugar, can contribute to cavities (because they stick to teeth, as well as because of their sugar content) and are contraindicated in hypoglycemia. Home-dried apples, peaches, and apricots, on the other hand, when reconstituted in water, may need a bit of honey for sweetening.

11

Outdoor Gardening

Outdoor gardening can be done on a large or small scale. If space is a problem, grow vegetables in containers. They must be watered and fertilized oftener, but resist pests better, particularly gophers and moles that gnaw away roots. Winter gardens can be grown outdoors by those who live in milder climates. Use hardy seeds such as beets, carrots, celery, Chinese cabbage, chives, chard, lettuce, kohlrabi, leeks, parsnips, peas and snow peas (edible pod), radishes, rutabaga, spinach and turnips. Set out plants of cabbage, cauliflower, brussels sprouts, lettuce and broccoli. A greenhouse or cold frame can be used by those who live in colder climates.

Indoor Gardening

Seed sprouting is the simplest method of getting fresh, raw food with high vitamin and mineral content year-round, in any climate. The sprouts can be used in salads, sandwiches, or just plain as snacks, particularly for children. There are many types of seed sprouters available but they are not really necessary. My lazy method is to soak the seeds overnight, then place a paper towel in a colander and arrange the seeds on it, one layer deep. Cover with another paper towel. Put the colander with seeds and towels under running water until the towels are soaking wet. Let them drain in the sink. Place out of the way in a corner of the kitchen counter until next day. Re-irrigate daily. Continue for two or three days until the seeds have sprouted approximately an inch. Store the sprouted seeds in the refrigerator. More vitamin and mineral content is retained if the sprouts are not cooked. If adding to soups or omelets, add at the last moment, so that they are warmed only.

The little green jackets of mung bean sprouts, too tough for some people to eat, can be floated away by putting the sprouts in a bowl full of water and agitating

12

the water. Wheat and rye sprouts should be short. They can become too stringy to eat.

Some seeds are grown indoors in soil for a supply of fresh greens. This is done by putting ⅝ of an inch of good soil in trays and planting wheat berries for wheat grass, whole sunflower seeds for greens (delicious) or buckwheat seeds for buckwheat lettuce, rich in rutin, as well as lecithin and chlorophyll.

Method of Indoor Gardening

1. Soak seeds overnight.
2. Put soil in trays and spread seeds on top of soil.
3. Place 8 layers of wet newspapers, topped with plastic, on seeds.
4. Remove covering when sprouts are 2½ inches high.
5. Place in sunlight until they are 6 inches high.
6. Cut and eat raw greens.

For further information on indoor gardening, see the Additional Reading list.

For sources of seeds (which must not be coated with poisons or fungicides) try health food stores or see the Special Supplies list (1). Quick-growing cress seed can be procured from seed companies.

Peace of Mind

Of utmost importance during an emergency survival crisis is your state of mind. Confidence and serenity are necessary for your own well-being as well as for the reassurance of those around you. Keep your sense of humor. Of what use is it to protect your bodies while you let your nerves blow? If you are panicky, irritated or resentful, keep thinking, "This, too, will pass. Tomorrow is another day."

A true story was brought back from Vietnam by a group of POWs. While they were confined as prisoners, they had nothing to do to keep up their morale, nothing to read, and little hope. One man began trying to remember comforting verses from the Bible. He could not remember all of the words of the biblical messages. He asked his cell mates. They, too, joined the game. Before long they were whispering through the walls of the next cell, and this was carried on to the next cell. Remembered verses were written on anything available—the floor and the wall. They were even written on toilet tissue and passed around. The men said it was the only type of constructive thinking available which freed them from worry. It literally, they said, kept their minds from blowing.

Finally, after many requests, the guards loaned them a Bible for reference work for one hour daily. Through prayer and contemplation on a power higher than their own, they survived.

One woman has her own recipe for survival. She says, "If you are lost in the woods, or caught in a survival crisis of *any* kind, there are three rules to follow: 1. Be calm. 2. Be calm. 3. Be calm."

General Supplies

- Warm clothing, socks, blankets, inexpensive survival blankets (from recreational suppliers), sleeping bags, plastic sheets, tarpaulins, hats, raincoats.
- Comfortable shoes for walking (there may be no gasoline for cars). Bicycles.
- Cooking equipment: camping stoves and appropriate fuel, Sterno (canned heat *must* have proper ventilation if used indoors) and Sterno folding stoves; charcoal for fireplace or barbecue cooking.
- Lighting: candles and holders, lanterns, flash-

lights, batteries, kerosene lamps and kerosene safely stored in metal, plastic or glass container.

- Wood for fireplaces. Matches stored in air-tight containers. Dip large matches in paraffin, store in closed containers. To light, remove a bit of wax with fingernail. The wax will protect against moisture or combustion and will burn longer and better than un-waxed matches.
- Non-electric equipment (in case of power failure): hand can opener, wind-up clock, transistor radio and batteries, juice can opener and hand egg-beater to replace blender.
- Paper products: tissues, toilet tissue, paper towels, plates, bowls, napkins and cups (all can be used for fuel later).
- Old pots and pans and kitchen cutlery, knives, forks; wide-mouth thermos for cooking grains; heavy-duty aluminum foil.
- Secondhand refrigerators for food storage. (Inexpensive when bought from Good Will or secondhand outlets. May be old but durable.) Store in basement or garage. If there is a power shortage, do not open these or freezers for forty-eight hours, at which time power may be restored.
- Heavy-duty plastic bags for human waste in case of water failure.
- Boxes and bags for garbage disposal (which may be temporarily discontinued). Put food scraps on compost heaps.
- Field glasses, hearing aid batteries and other special needs, shaving equipment, sanitary napkins, disposable diapers and baby oil for babies.
- Mending equipment: needle, scissors, assorted thread and thimble.

- Beauty needs: cleansing cream, hand cream, nail file, hand mirror, etc.
- Liquid soap, biodegradable.
- Toothbrush (toothpaste not necessary) and dental floss.
- First aid supplies: Band-Aids, iodine, chlorophyll, cloves and oil of cloves for toothache, tweezers for thorn removal, cotton, rubbing alcohol.
- Water storage and water purifying supplies.
- Time passers: paper and pen, playing cards, games and musical instruments.
- Reading material: all those books you have always meant to read, along with such favorites as the Bible.

Special Supplies

1. Available through The Survival Service, from Comfort Products Co., P.O. Box 742, Soquel, Cal. 95073. Write for free catalog.
2. A lifetime supply of active kefir grains can be ordered from R-A-J Biological Laboratory, 35 Park Ave., Blue Point, N.Y. 11715.
3. Grains, seeds and flours are available from health stores, Walnut Acres, Penns Creek, Pa. 17862 or The Survival Service.
4. Write for information to Ann Wigmore, D.D., N.D., Hippocrates Health Institute, 25 Exeter St., Boston, Mass. 02116.
5. For dehydrated food, write Pro-Vita Foods, 1425 Ft. Lincoln Ave., Anaheim, Cal. 92805.

Additional Reading

Robert L. Preston. *How to Prepare for the Coming Crash.* Salt Lake City, Utah: Hawkes Publishing, 1971.

This book shows you how to prepare for and live through the possible coming depression predicted by Mr. Preston, an economist, writer and lecturer. It also contains suggestions for surviving power failures, food and service strikes, prolonged unemployment and illness, floods, earthquakes, tornadoes, hurricanes, etc. Interesting and easy to read. A must.

Esther Dickey. *Passport to Survival.* New York, N.Y.: Random House, 1974.
A complete and excellent book to help you plan and store your survival program.

Mike Samuels, M.D. and Hal Bennett. *The Well Body Book.* Berkeley, Cal.: Bookworks, 1973.
A book to help you keep well at any time. Very popular.

Gen MacManiman. *Dry It—You'll Like It!* Seattle, Wash.: Montana Books, 1974.
An excellent book about dehydrating food, including recipes and plans for building your own dehydrator.

Beatrice Trum Hunter. *Fact Book on Yogurt, Kefir and Other Milk Cultures.* Also, *Fact Book on Fermented Foods and Beverages.* New Canaan, Conn.: Keats Publishing, both 1973.
Everything you need to know about making cultured milk products and fermented foods.

J. B. Chapman, M.D. *Dr. Schuessler's Biochemistry.* J. W. Cogswell, ed. St. Louis, Mo.: Formur International, 1975.
A small, wonderful book to explain cell salts and their uses for various ailments.

Ken and Pat Kraft. *Growing Food the Natural Way.* New York, N.Y.: Doubleday, 1973.
One of the best books on organic gardening.

Charles Morrow Wilson. *Let's Try Barter: The answer to inflation and the tax collector.* Old Greenwich, Conn.: Devin-Adair Co., 1960.
A charming book which may be the answer to the problem of devalued money. As Robert Preston says, "Barter works! My father bought a new car during the 1929 depression for five hundred pounds of potatoes." Many

other examples of barter are in this book. The book should eventually pay for itself.

Stuart Wheelwright *Plan and Survive.*
A helpful little book including information on foods, natural first aid remedies, recipes, seed sprouting.

Ann Wigmore, D.D., N.D. *Indoor Organic Gardening.* Hippocrates Health Institute, 25 Exeter St., Boston, Mass. 02116.

Which Reducing Diet Is Best?

ONE OF THE NATION'S leading experts on obesity believes that there is not a single cause of obesity in all people, but that a multiplicity of factors and an interrelationship of these factors can cause overweight.

I would add that although there are some common denominators, there are also individual differences. Just because you and your friend next door are both ten pounds overweight does not necessarily mean that the reasons are the same, or that the same kind of diet will work for you both.

Before you choose a diet that will work for you (and there should be one that does), some honest analysis of your problem—not that of your neighbor or even others in your family—should help you to pick the best reducing diet for you.

So let's look at the individual problems first and discuss the common denominators later. Spot-check the following problems in order to find your own.

What Is the Size of Your Frame?

Age-height-weight tables are not absolutely reliable. Some take into account the size of your frame; others do not. If you have a larger-than-average frame and heavier bones, obviously your weight will be influenced. You may be overweight according to the chart, but not fat. A reducing diet is not for you.

What Is Your Genetic Inheritance?

Genes are a factor. Dr. Jean Mayer states that certain animals have a tendency to put on more weight than others, even though their diet is identical with animals which are not overweight. If your parents and grandparents tended toward fat, it may be a genetic inheritance, or it may be that the love for fat-producing food runs in the family. The German diet, for example, usually produces more corpulence than the Scandinavian diet. Because of national inheritances, some foods agree better with some people than with others.

The Scandinavians have thrived on seafood for generations. The Italians, living in their warm, sunny climate, thrive on fruits and vegetables. Orientals have subsisted on refined rice for centuries with no noticeable effects, whereas others find it a nutritionally inadequate food.

Your body type is another consideration. Some types naturally gain weight more easily than others. If you are one of these, your eating must, of course, differ from those who can eat anything they wish without gaining.

What About Your Metabolism?

You have heard again and again the advice, "Consult your doctor before going on a reducing diet." There are two good reasons for this. One reason is that there are physical disturbances which can cause overweight. Although they affect only a minority of overweight people, they are often the cause in the extremely fat person. Extreme obesity may be traced to glandular imbalance, dysfunction of the brain center regulating food intake, or a metabolic disturbance. In the latter case, the fat person may not digest or assimilate his food properly. Digestive enzymes may help here. The doctor can help to establish the cause of such physical disturbances.

I know of one couple in different metabolic categories.

The man has been greatly overweight until recently (a doctor spotted his problem and helped him trim down). His wife, who actually eats more than he does, remains a svelte size eight.

Another reason for a doctor's supervision is to prevent the use of dangerous fad diets, which I will discuss later.

Do You Get Enough Exercise?

Dr. Mayer believes that the greatest cause of overweight is inactivity. Research proves this to be true with animals, as every farmer already knows. Dr. Mayer believes that a combination of self-indulgence and lack of exercise can cause overweight. He and others deplore the on-again, off-again dieting which he terms "the rhythm method of girth control." It has been found to throw out of kilter the glandular machinery for regulating body functions. The glands become so confused by the constant changes that their efficiency finally breaks down. Avoid see-saw dieting.

Are You Habit Bound?

Many people are accustomed to eating large amounts of food. Their stomachs have stretched and constantly demand the same amount. A woman on a Weight-Watcher's diet was weighing her food portions according to instructions. She had a little bit left over. Before she realized it, she had popped it into her mouth out of habit. The children who were taught to "clean up your plate" are still doing it as adults.

Queen Elizabeth of England is an example of what good eating habits can do. When she was married, her waist measured twenty-six inches. Her family tends to overweight (witness her plump mother and plumpish sister). The Queen at first followed this pattern and became matronly and overweight. Then she changed her eating habits (with the help of a doctor) and today her waist measures two inches less than at the time of her marriage, even though she is fiftyish and the mother of four children. Her secret is not a diet, but smaller helpings. She has learned to become a small eater.

So try the simplest method of losing weight: use the eat-just-half plan; chew that half well; enjoy it. Your stomach may be used to more food and argue for increased amounts, but if you can stick it out for three or four days, your stomach will shrink and you have it made!

Are You a Gulper?

Fat people usually gulp their food. Often they are not even aware of what they are eating or what it tastes like. Horace Fletcher invented the fine art of chewing thoroughly. If you Fletcherize—chew each bite until it is liquified—you will get more satisfaction from your food, eat less, digest it better and normalize weight.

Do You Live to Eat?

People who live alone or who feel sorry for themselves often stuff themselves. Although it is true that some elderly people living alone "eat like birds" because they hate to cook for only one person, other single retirees have no other interest. Their first thought when they get up in the morning is "What shall I eat today?"

Rewarding yourself with food for bad luck, rejection, lack of love, appreciation or attention from other people, or because of other emotional disturbances, is one of the easiest ways to gain weight. One woman, a successful wife and mother, had really enjoyed her role in life. She was a former model, beautiful, with a perfect figure. She was admired by all, including her husband. Because of circumstances beyond her control, her husband left her. She lost interest in her appearance, ate constantly to forget her grief and now looks like a stuffed pincushion. Her interest in her children also waned. Had she not given in to psychologically negative influences she could have had her choice of suitors, but she has lost all interest in life except eating for consolation.

Finding a new interest to replace self-pity—perhaps doing something to help others—would solve the problem for both the lonely retired person and anyone living in an emotional vacuum.

Have You Given Up Smoking?

Smoking is another substitute satisfaction when someone is suffering from stress, insecurity or ragged nerves. It is also a habit. Many people who give up smoking eat sweets or overeat to compensate, but the resulting weight gain is only temporary. When you give up smoking the body eventually adjusts, you feel better and your metabolism improves, finally resulting in normal weight.

Do You Have Hidden Hunger?

Many people overeat because they are always hungry. One reason for this is that their bodies are not getting the nutrients they need or crave. In this era of empty calories, of refined and processed foods, it may take a lot of these foods to supply the body's needs. A woman once told me she craved bread and ate it, slice after slice. Her weight soared. When she began making her own bread of whole grains and other body-satisfying nutrients, one slice of bread satisfied her. Her weight dropped as her hidden hunger disappeared.

Are You a Water Storer?

Some people are overweight, not because they are fat, but because they store water, become bloated and appear fat, particularly in some parts of their body, such as abdomen or ankles. If this edema is caused by heart trouble, obviously you should consult a doctor, who may advise a diuretic to rid the body of water. But for reducing purposes, beware of diuretic drugs! In one reducing clinic maintained by an M.D., I was shocked to learn that diuretic drugs are routinely prescribed for all who come to the clinic to reduce.

One person told me she was given a diuretic drug at bedtime and that she spent the night racing to the bathroom. By morning, she had lost seven pounds and was so weak she could scarcely walk. Worst of all, with this sudden flushing of water from her body went all the B vitamins and other water-soluble nutrients. There are safer diuretics, including herbal diuretics, vitamin C in large doses, vitamin B-6 and minerals.

John M. Ellis, M.D., found during his years of research that 50 mgs of vitamin B-6 daily helped rid menopausal and premenstrual women of excess water; even men ranchers were able to tighten their belts to the last notch without going on a reducing diet at all. Salt (sodium chloride) is said to be one factor in causing water storage. Potassium helps to counteract this storage. Dr. Ellis learned that vitamin B-6 apparently helps to set up the proper balance or ratio between sodium and potassium, which regulate body fluids. Magnesium has been found helpful in some cases, too. Taking a vitamin supplement with a complete source of easily assimilated minerals, plus vitamin B-6, is far safer than a diuretic drug for gradual elimination of excess water from the body.

Do You Take Reducing Drugs?

Watch it! Reports indicate that reducing drugs, including appetite depressants, may increase the pulse rate and cause shakiness in some people. Henry Brill, M.D., states: "Over-use can result in excessive beating of the heart, high blood pressure, nervousness, emotional tension, even hallucinations."

James B. Landis, of a well-known drug company, warns that even pep pills can affect the appetite center of the brain and may cause a psychosis similar to schizophrenia.

The American Medical Association warns that diet pills, including thyroid, hormones, digitalis and diuretics, may not work and can be dangerous. At least sixty deaths have resulted from taking diet pills.

Is Reducing an Obsession with You?

Many women try to look like the somewhat emaciated models in the chic fashion magazines. Unlike those people who are compulsive eaters, some women go to the other extreme and are obsessed by compulsive reducing. These unfortunates weigh daily, and if they gain a pound or even less (weight can fluctuate temporarily in either direction without being serious), these women panic. I know three of them. They can think of little else. They feel guilt-ridden when they eat. Such people can make themselves and their families miserable.

If you can't get into a dress you wore twenty years ago because you have changed an inch or so in your measurements, forget it! Childbirth, even improved nutrition, can make some changes in your dimensions and this may be a sign you are either normal for your age, or even better than you were twenty years ago.

Salvator Cutolo, M.D., believes that many people should not be thin. He feels it is better to be a little overweight, even as much as ten pounds. Although excessive weight is to be discouraged for reasons of both health and appearance, Dr. Cutolo believes that a small surplus of weight gives you a reserve of energy if you should need it, and that women who are emaciated or too thin are more nervous and harder to live with.

I am sure both husbands and children would prefer wives and mothers to be a few pounds overweight and cheerful and relaxed, to being women who make a fetish of being thin and snap irritably at their families because of their reducing obsession. Life is too short. Decide which is more important.

Which Reducing Diet Is Best?

Now, having determined whether your trouble may be physical, emotional or psychological in origin, or caused by inactivity or genetic conditions, the wrong food, or a combination of these factors, what do you do about it?

Dr. Jean Mayer says, "A 'good' reducing diet is one in which the patient does not become too hungry." I say that a good reducing diet should also be a way of life, not a state of panic. It should provide all the nutrients the body needs for health and be simple and satisfying for *you* so that once you have planned and adopted it, you can turn your attention to other things. It should not be a goal in itself, but a means to a better life.

Fasting

Fasting, at least total fasting on water alone, can be suicidal and I mean just that. Those who point out that fasting dates back to biblical days and gets all the poisons out of the body to produce good health, forget that we are not living in biblical times. Today we are living in a totally different environment of polluted air, water and food. For instance, the DDT we have picked up along the way is stored in our fatty tissues. During total (water only) fasting, these poisons are released suddenly into our bloodstream as the fat breaks down, and so we poison ourselves.

Fasting has led to illness, even death, within the last few years. Even a one-sided diet of one single good food, continued too long, has proved dangerous. A young housewife told me that she had gone on such a diet for several weeks without taking supplements to supply the missing factors her body needed, and nearly died. A short fast of juices or a single food used for a few days only, or supervised by a physician if used longer—provided that all known supplements are used—can help to cleanse the body safely.

Dr. Mayer says that fasting will, indeed, cause a weight loss, but this loss will be protein, not fat, and cause the muscles to melt away. Four physicians at the University of California studied eleven obese patients on a prolonged water fast, plus vitamin pills. Serious complications developed in every one of the cases. The conditions included anemia, low blood pressure and gout. The problems disappeared when the patients resumed eating.

Fad Diets

Fad diets are nutritionally inadequate. They may consist of one or more foods, such as bananas or rice. One physician and one dentist told me that many illnesses in their patients began with fad diets. To be healthy, the body needs at least sixty nutrients *every day*. One single food *cannot* contain them all. Prisoners of war, restricted to one or a few foods, developed deficiencies from which they never recovered. Dr. Robert McCarrison, the late internationally respected nutritionist, found during his lifetime study of nutritional effects on animals that all organs suffer when they are deprived of proper nutrition.

Fat-Free Diets

A fat-free diet is a snake in the grass. Many women shun fat as if it were poison. Many men shun it because their doctors told them to stay away from cholesterol.

27

Many doctors warn their patients that a high-fat diet will cause heart trouble.

The body cannot assimilate the fat-soluble vitamins (A, B, E and K) without fat. The intestines cannot manufacture B vitamins without fat, particularly linoleic acid, an unsaturated oil. Wilfrid E. Shute, M.D., points out that our forefathers ate animal fats, ate fried foods in abundance and did not trim their meat, yet there is no record of coronary thrombosis before the year 1911, shortly after vitamin E was milled out of our grain, cereals, and bread. He says that to consider fat the major cause of heart disease is a *myth*. It is true that moderation, not complete elimination of fat in the diet, is recommended.

Adelle Davis told the story of a model who tried everything to lose weight; nothing worked until she took two or more tablespoons of oil daily. Hair and skin lose luster on a fat-free diet. Gallstones have been traced to a fat-free diet. And as you add more unsaturated oil to your diet, you need more vitamin E to balance it. There is more than one book, written by an M.D., that shows one can grow slim by adding some fat to the diet. A medium- or low-fat diet is safer than a no-fat diet. Furthermore, it keeps you from getting so hungry.

As for avoiding cholesterol, this is out of date. The body manufactures cholesterol whether you eat it or not, and many glands, including sex glands, need cholesterol for proper maintenance. Adding lecithin to the diet has been found by Dr. Lester Morrison, as well as Adelle Davis and other nutritionists, to be far more effective in lowering cholesterol than cutting out valuable foods that contain cholesterol.

The Low-Calorie Diet

Calorie-counting is now out of date. Bernard A. Bellew, M.D., states that this method is inaccurate and fallible. Dr. Richard Mackarness says, "It does not work for the majority of overweights." The *American Journal of Clinical Nutrition* agrees (1).

The Nibble Diet

The nibble diet is a method of eating in which the same amount of food formerly eaten during three square meals a day is redistributed into six or more small, frequent meals. Ben Weider, the health and exercise expert, has stated that by including high-protein foods, fresh green vegetables and a little fruit each day, with a minimum of bread, one can lose weight, feel better and avoid hunger on the nibble diet. He says, "After I was on this diet for ten days, I lost four pounds and never once felt the pangs of hunger. At suppertime I ate a hot meal along with the rest of the family, but I ate very little of everything."

A study of 450 men revealed that those who ate two big meals daily gained more weight than those who ate four or five meals per day. The reason: A smaller amount of food is easier to digest and can be burned up quickly instead of being stored as fat, report the researchers of this study. According to a study at New York State University Medical Center, small, frequent meals are also considered to have a better effect on the heart and other organs and tissues; metabolism and assimilation improve. Dr. Mayer adds that this method can lower high cholesterol.

A nibble diet is also a boon for hypoglycemics (sufferers from low blood sugar).

The New York State researchers warn against heavy and late evening meals, one of the greatest sources of overweight.

The Low Carbohydrate Diet

Not all diets work for all people. The diet prescribed for the overweight man with the size eight wife, mentioned earlier, consisted of no sugar, flour or alcohol, and temporarily no fat or dairy products except for skim-milk cheese. He was allowed unlimited fresh fruits, vegetables, white meat of chicken and fish, plus vitamins E and C, and homeopathic substances. He lost forty-five pounds in two months and feels wonderful. But this does not mean it is *your* solution. It was planned by a doctor for this man alone.

The grapefruit diet is another questionable reducing diet. This is basically a high-protein diet with a half grapefruit or a glass of grapefruit juice to be taken before each meal. I have seen some people lose weight on it, whereas others lost nary an ounce. It can be dynamite for arthritics who have learned that citrus fruit intensifies their symptoms and pain, or for those who are allergic to citrus fruit.

The one diet that seems to be successful for more people than any other is the low-carbohydrate diet. It deserves your full attention and is definitely worth a fair and prolonged trial. It not only helps most people reduce, but helps them stay healthy. Carbohydrates are mainly starches and sweets. Excess carbohydrates are stored as fat in the body (and flabby fat at that). Protein, on the other hand, feeds muscles and makes them firm. Carbohydrates have also been implicated in tooth decay, heart disease and fatigue.

William I. Kauffman, popular author, stated that he had watched his weight for twenty-five years and the low-carbohydrate diet is the only one that really worked for him. One does not need to become hungry on this diet. Some people even find they need smaller servings and fewer than sixty grams of carbohydrates.

The theory of the low-carbohydrate diet is that by eating sixty grams or less of carbohydrates per day, fat in the body is burned up, not stored. There is no limit to calories (you will find some surprises, believe me) and the diet restricts carbohydrates only. It is easy, fun and rewarding. Scientific studies galore confirm its success in reducing weight.

Fresh raw fruit may be eaten freely even though high in carbohydrate count. Man-made carbohydrates, including pies, cakes, cookies and other starches and sweets are the pound-gainers. Some foods are in between, to be used with caution.

One section of my book *Be Slim and Healthy* (2) is a list of foods in the form of a Go-Caution-Stop Carbohydrate Computer. Sample entries: Apples, 1 large raw = 27.3 grams, G; Apple brown betty, ½ c. = 35.2 grams, S; Apple butter, 1 Tbs. = 8.5 grams, C. The Go-Caution-Stop computer is also available separately, in a size you can carry along with you in your purse or pocket (3).

Any diet should be combined with nutritional supplements for health insurance, and the low carbohydrate diet is no exception.

Dr. Bellew says you can even go on an eating binge now and then on this diet and still stay slim. So give it a try.

References

1. *American Journal of Clinical Nutrition.* March 1971.
2. Linda Clark. *Be Slim and Healthy.* New Canaan, Conn.: Keats Publishing, 1972.
3. Linda Clark. *Go-Caution-Stop Carbohydrate Computer.* New Canaan, Conn.: Keats Publishing, 1973.

Safe Drinking Water

IN THESE DAYS of polluted water, the old saying "Water, water everywhere and not a drop to drink" describes the dilemma that is developing around us. Not only is tap water unacceptable in many localities, but also wells and mountain streams which formerly yielded delicious, clean and healthful water are now unpleasant to taste and smell and may be a threat to health. Tap water and wells can harbor impurities from home and factory wastes (which have killed fish in large numbers) and can also collect impurities from the seepage of tanks and cesspools in overdeveloped living areas. In less crowded farm communities they can pick up the drainage of pesticides used in home gardening as well as barnyard drainage.

Detergents are still another threat. For example, in New Mexico on Monday mornings, the drinking water supply of a small town about thirty miles south of Albuquerque has been reported to be suddenly filled with billowing suds as a result of the detergents used in washing machines.

That delightful spring water our forefathers used to drink from the family tin cup hanging by the well or spring is no longer with us. Water in formerly fresh mountain streams and springs has been tested and found to contain a variety of pollutants. One of the greatest hazards is lead, which is sucked up into the atmosphere from car exhausts, widely distributed by winds and eventually deposited in soil and water by air, rain and snow.

Even drinking water flowing through pipes of various metals from municipal water supplies can be contaminated by lead, mercury, cadmium and excessive copper— all toxic substances—and delivered right to your own home and into your drinking glass.

No wonder people are becoming panicky! Where can we find safe water to drink? Fortunately there are a few hopeful solutions to the problem, as well as some hazards to avoid.

Bottled Water

Just because water is bought in a bottle does not insure its safety. Fortunately, there is an American Bottled Water Association to which 90 percent of the water bottlers belong; they voluntarily impose their own regulatory standards. As an example, for a long time I had bought commercial bottled water, taken from a mountain spring and labeled "Pure Spring Water." One day, however, I noticed the driver had left a bottle with a different label: "Spring Fresh Water." On checking with the company I was told that they could no longer stand behind the label of "Pure Spring Water." Analysis of the water showed contamination, they said. The substitute, "Spring Fresh Water," was actually a distilled water to which the company had added some (but not all) minerals.

Since distillation removes all minerals as well as contaminants, I asked the chemist for the water company if there were other methods of water purification. He answered, "There are three methods: distillation, reversed osmosis, and deionization."

I also asked the water chemist if we were better off with distilled water with added minerals than with natural spring water. He said, "I would not drink most natural spring water any longer. If you could see an analysis of such water today, it would frighten you." He explained that every stream, every spring large enough to supply many people (perhaps even just a few) is now polluted. Then he made a surprising statement: "But if one is drinking straight distilled water, that person *must* get added minerals from his diet or from mineral supplements, because the distilled water will leach minerals from his body."

Not everyone agrees with this statement from an honest water chemist. However, it becomes a clue, as I will explain later, to safe drinking water.

In comparison with such commercial honesty, I have heard unconfirmed rumors that a few dealers sell ordinary tap water in bottles. In 1973, the Food and Drug Administration proposed some regulatory standards to cope with this problem. When eighty-five different brands of bottled water were tested, eight were found to contain coliform bacteria from human waste as well as excessive levels of copper and lead.

There is still one brand of bottled water that comes from a highly protected natural spring in Arkansas which is considered safe. It has been in use for over a century. Many United States presidents have used it, even taking it with them when travelling.

The analyses of this water, taken thirty years apart, show unusual constancy. The spring is covered with a dome to prevent contamination from the air, and the water is drawn off below the surface level to prevent ground contamination. The water is shipped to most states and the price reflects the distance and transportation costs from the bottling source. One of its advantages is that it has a pH (acidity rating) of 7.6 which helps to assure the assimilation of beneficial minerals. It is called Mountain Valley Water and comes from Arkansas.

Fluoridated Water

There have been reams of material published, pro and con, as to the dangers or benefits of fluoridated water. I will merely give you the essence of what I have learned.

The types of fluorides added to city water supplies are identified as poisons. According to John J. Miller, Ph.D., a biochemist, the fluorides have been found to interfere with thirty-one known enzymes critically important to health and life. The dangerous effects have a delayed reaction and many dentists who originally recommended their use in dentistry are changing their opinions.

One of the most serious aspects of fluorides in a city water supply is that they are distributed unevenly, piling up in greater concentration in some areas, giving a too-high dosage to people with kidney disease who cannot effectively liberate poisons from their bodies. The sensible approach would be for a doctor to prescribe fluorides for those who might need them, rather than mass-drugging the entire population via the water systems (1).

If you wish further information, write to the Pure Water Association of America, P.O. Box 424, Berkeley, California 94701.

Chlorinated Water

Chlorinated water is the easiest water problem to solve. To remove the unpleasant odor and taste from highly chlorinated tap water, boil it for a few minutes and cool before refrigerating, or allow it to stand in an open container overnight. In either case, the chlorine evaporates and is completely dissipated.

Purifying Water at Home

There are many devices available which promise to "purify" your water. They may indeed remove some contaminants but not all. Or they remove everything—

35

minerals, as well as contaminants—leaving a lifeless or inert liquid. One company, for example, manufactures a charcoal filtering device which claims to "instantly remove chlorine, sulphur, metallics, rust, scale and algae from drinking water." There are many contaminants not mentioned. (Incidentally, no device is allowed to claim removal of fluorides, even if true.)

There is one unique filter, relatively inexpensive if compared with the more costly distillers, which contains some natural mineral deposits through which the tap water runs. The device attaches quickly to the water tap and decontaminates as well as remineralizes water which, after refrigeration, has a delicious flavor similar to the old-time pure mountain streams. I have tested it and like it.*

Softened Water

Deionizing water is one method of removing minerals from water with, for instance, a water softener. By running the hard water through salt, the other minerals are attracted away from the water and drawn off. This is why so many who feel that they must have soft water for laundry and dishwashing purposes do not have their cold water—used for beverages or cooking—attached to the water softener. They do not want to lose the valuable health-giving minerals.

Water softened by artificial water softeners, according to the University of California Agricultural Extension Service, should *not* be drunk since it contains so much salt (sodium) from the softening process.

Distilled Water

There is raging controversy being waged over distilled water. Those who defend it insist it is the *only* pure

---

*For information, write Shali-Min of New Mexico, Inc., 1605 Coal Avenue, S.E., Albuquerque, New Mexico 87106.

water. This may be true, but you can be sure it is also water which has had all the nutrients (minerals) removed along with the contaminants. You will recall that the water chemist mentioned earlier warned that distilled water would leach the minerals from the body. Since health is dependent upon minerals, the practice of distillation can create an extremely serious health situation, except possibly for short-term use.

Inorganic Minerals

A few writers frighten the public by stating that you should not drink hard water because it contains inorganic minerals. They cite a few isolated cases as proof that these minerals can pile up in the body causing calcium and other deposits, resulting in arthritis, atherosclerosis (hardening of the arteries), a rare condition of "turning to stone" due to the deposit of minerals in the tissues, as well as heart disease. It is *never* safe to generalize! Scientific tests the world over do not support those who are pushing the panic button about inorganic minerals or hard water that contains various minerals.

As proof that hard water (which contains more minerals than soft or than distilled water with none at all) does *not* necessarily cause heart disease, an experiment with New Zealand rabbits showed that those which drank hard water had *less* heart disease than those which drank distilled water(2).

Henry A. Schroeder, M.D., of Dartmouth Medical School, perhaps one of the world's most knowledgeable experts on minerals, reported in 1960 that fewer people die of heart disease in areas where the water is relatively hard than in areas where the water is soft. This finding applied to both England and the United States(3). There is now general confirmation(4).

Scientists of W.H.O. (World Health Organization) also have found through extensive research that areas using soft water have a greater occurrence of heart attacks than do populations using hard water. They believe that the minerals in the hard water, particularly calcium, are responsible for the heart protection. *Distilled water, they report, is 100 percent soft* (5). (Emphasis mine.)

The human body *must* have minerals; it is made of minerals and as they are used up daily to maintain health, they must also be replaced daily. Water should be one universal source of these minerals, as nature intended. Otherwise, trouble can result. For example, in Europe a while back some athletes started a cross-country run, announcing that they would consume nothing but distilled water for a number of days while completing their trek. A little more than halfway to their announced goal they were forced to discontinue drinking the distilled water. All had lost so much of their mineral reserves, including the vitally important electrolytes, that had they continued with their plan it could have proved very serious, even fatal(6).

One expert, who lives in one of the largest cities in this country, wrote me: "On spending an entire day at our county medical association library and questioning doctors at our local health department on the subject of distilled water leaching the minerals from the body, one of the doctors verified the dangers of mineral leaching and even stated that a person could actually die as a result of drinking only distilled water for an extended period of time.

"An article stated that water with too few minerals [soft water] eats up the plumbing, so imagine what it would do to human plumbing. Still another article showed that rats given *tap* water for four weeks showed the least damage, whereas those given *distilled* water were the most damaged. All but two [of these] died."

Dr. Hazel Parcells, Ph.D., a nutritionist, says, "We

found that using distilled water, as well as water from water softeners, for drinking and cooking, caused definite muscle weakness, the heart being one of the first victims of this poor mineral balance. Also the general muscle tone throughout the body was very poor. The blood chemistry of these people showed a low calcium and a deficiency of other supportive minerals."

A reader wrote me, "After reading a book on drinking water, my husband insists on drinking distilled water. All it has done for him is to give him a sore knee, a sore elbow and terrific pains between the shoulder blades. When we went on our vacation we used only well water, and he never had a pain all the time we were gone. Still, I cannot convince him that he needs water which contains all the minerals rather than water which has had them removed. I have also read that more heart attacks occur where the water is soft (low in minerals) than where it is hard (high in minerals). I love my husband too much to have him become a candidate for a heart attack."

Why do some people develop arthritis, hardening of the arteries and other problems when they drink so-called hard water containing calcium and other minerals? It is extremely important to realize that it may not be the fault of the *water* with its minerals, but the *person* who drinks the water. Calcium and iron cannot be dissolved in water or even in the body *without some acid*. If you do not believe this, drop a hard calcium tablet in a glass of water or milk. The chances are that it will not dissolve or disintegrate. But if you add some apple cider vinegar to the water, the calcium will break up! Dr. D. C. Jarvis reported that farm animals with arthritic symptoms recovered when acid (vinegar) was added to their drinking water. Dr. Jarvis also found that vinegar dissolves the mineral deposits coating the inside of a tea kettle.

Many authorities agree that if the body lacks hydrochloric acid for proper digestion, or is deficient in vitamin C (another form of acid), neither iron nor calcium can be dissolved and kept in solution, but apparently are laid down in unwanted deposits. Now, you will remember that the Arkansas natural spring water, that contains all minerals, has a pH (acidity rating) of 7.6. The slight acidity helps the body to digest and assimilate the minerals. The human skin and hair—if healthy—also have a pH of 7.6. Good health is dependent on this acidity.

So let us not jump to hasty conclusions and blame hard, mineral-rich water for some diseases, when their cause is actually a lack in the person and not the water. Above all, don't blame the inorganic minerals. Both inorganic and organic minerals are needed by the body. On autopsy, the inorganic minerals are found in the ashes of a healthy body. If there is a deficiency of any of these minerals, organic or inorganic, health becomes disturbed. J. B. Chapman, M.D., says: "The human body is composed of two kinds of matter, organic and inorganic ... indeed the organic could not perform its proper function without the inorganic."

The late esteemed Dr. William A. Albrecht, Professor Emeritus of Soils, College of Agriculture, University of Missouri, said, "We have too long believed that the nutritious inorganic elements from the soils must be water-soluble. Some insoluble (inorganic) substances, on coming in contact with the mucous membrane of the body, become soluble and harmless there."

The Hunzas are proof that water containing inorganic minerals is a source of health. Betty Morales and John T. Clark, after returning from Hunzaland wrote, "The Hunzas are a remote people living high in the Karakorum chain of mountains, in Kashmir, Pakistan. Hunza has only about three inches of rainfall annually, and thus must bring water for crops and domestic use from glacial peaks reaching more than 20,000 feet high, where snows and ice are eternal, never completely melting. This water is carried in stone-lined ditches. When viewed in a glass it is milky in appearance. Even after settling for a week, the minerals do not precipitate out: thus they are colloidal in nature, from constant friction, particle against particle, against rock.

"Crops irrigated with this highly mineralized water do not attract insects; history shows that soil fertility has been maintained for at least 2,300 years, since the time Alexander the Great came that way; and there has never been a single case of cancer in Hunza! Neither are there other degenerative diseases, although sanitation, as we know it, does not exist, and there are no drugs or hospitals.

"Ask the King of Hunza—called The Mir—why his people have such good health, strong teeth, good eyesight and enjoy a life expectancy of ninety years or more and he will tell you (as he did us when we were there) that first among the reasons is the *highly mineralized water*.

"Remember that nature produces no distilled water. Even rainwater, which is soft and nearly mineral-free, is not distilled; yet when used as the main source of potable water it can cause serious deficiencies, including heart trouble. Compare the minerals found in sea water and human blood; they are almost identical (7)."

This final remark brings us to the crux of the matter of finding a solution—water which is free from contaminants but helps supply the body with minerals. It is apparently not enough to drink distilled water and add minerals to your diet, because of the possible leaching action of distilled water.

The solution, then, is to add a balanced supply of *all* minerals to water so that it will *not* leach out or steal minerals from the body. The best way to do this is to add some sea water to your drinking water in proper proportions.

You may ask, "But, doesn't the United States Public Health Service warn against salt (sodium) content in drinking water because of edema?" (Edema is swelling caused by stored water in the body as a result of excessive retention of sodium by the kidneys.) Many (not all) doctors advocate a low sodium diet for this condition. What these health advisers are talking about is *sodium chloride, which is one factor only, not whole natural sea salt, or natural sea water*. Natural sea water contains major minerals and at least forty-four trace minerals in tiny amounts.

All minerals are needed for health and life. Sea water, when analyzed, is so similar to human blood analysis that doctors, in emergencies, have actually substituted sea water for blood in transfusions with excellent results. If all of these minerals are not present in aquarium sea water, or the aquarium sea water is synthetic, fish cannot live in it.

No doubt you, too, have already heard the following story that I had heard but never been able to confirm. To my delight, in 1972 I received a letter from a chemist connected with a Massachusetts marine laboratory. The letter read:

"Back around 1930 the aquarium in Chicago decided to make up sea water instead of having to bring it in tank cars from the Eastern coast. No matter how carefully they followed the chemical formula they had for sea water, it didn't work on the experimental fish they tried it on. The fish died.

"I was teaching science at a school in New York at the time. So I had several students try the same experiment. Again, failure. There are apparently traces of something or other that the analyses cannot catch. I imagine that even with the more exact spectroscopic analysis possible today the same thing would happen. In other words, sea water *has* something!"

In order to replace the minerals lost in distilled water, I asked a laboratory to devise a replacement formula using a small amount of natural sea water to produce a correct balance of minerals in drinking water. The flavor is palatable, particularly after the corrected water is refrigerated. I urge you not to dip up your own sea water from the edge of the shore, since most ocean water so close to land is contaminated by sewage. There is a natural, filtered, unheated source of sea water available in health stores, which has been taken from deep seas and is safe.

If you buy a distiller, I suggest that you get one made of stainless steel, since a test of one made of aluminum proved that it introduced aluminum into the water. In addition to adding the sea water to your drinking water, it is also wise to add extra minerals to your diet, either in foods or supplement form. At the end of this chapter I will give you the sea water-fortified formula, which you can make in your own home for safe drinking water. First, however, I want to give you some reassurance that sea water is safe to use. George W. Crane, Ph.D., M.D., has long recommended sea water in his syndicated newspaper column, "The Worry Clinic," for numerous health disturbances, not because sea water is a panacea, but because it helps the body to remedy mineral deficiencies which can lead to many disturbances. One of Dr. Crane's stories was about his father-in-law, a victim of arthritis.

"Eli Miller, aged ninety-seven, is Mrs. Crane's father, and is now taking one teaspoonful of sea water every day.

"After having been a chair patient for almost a year, during which time we had to lift him in and out of bed and often feed him by hand, he began to perk up.

"After he had spent four months on the sea brine treatment, I was mowing the lawn late one afternoon. As I passed the kitchen windows, I saw Grandpa Miller hobbling around with his aluminum walker. Please remember that he had been bedfast or chair-fast and was heading into his ninety-seventh birthday. If any changes were to occur, it would be natural to expect Grandpa to continue growing more feeble and more senile, wouldn't it?

"But he began to perk up, both mentally and physically. He now would get up unaided in the morning and put on his clothes. Then he'd walk to the bathroom and wash, after which he'd come to the table.

"The following night, Mrs. Crane motioned for me to come to his bedroom door and peek in. What I saw was the greatest miracle as regards his rejuvenation. For he had had an arthritic right hip for over ten years. When we'd dress him, he'd yell if we moved his right leg even gently. In fact, if his dog would accidentally bump that right leg, Grandpa would yell so you could hear him a block away.

"But now he lifted the arthritic right leg, crossed the right ankle over his left knee, and removed his shoe and sock; then let the right foot drop back upon the floor without letting out a peep! And if you had been around him for the past twenty years, as Mrs. Crane and I have, you'd realize that some miracle must have happened to his arthritic right hip!

"That was when I began to check back to see how we might explain his rejuvenation. And the *only* new item in his food or drink has been the daily teaspoon of sea water. (This one was concentrated ten times the usual ocean strength.)"

A reader wrote telling me that sea water had helped her arthritis and her insomnia as well. Her physician, she added, had refused to believe it at first, but became intrigued at her improvement as a result of using sea water.

A final story was told by Lee Hall, who has a Ph.D. in physiology. He says, "About eleven years ago a marine professor emeritus from Cal Tech, named George MacGinitie, was working for me on a special project to preserve the environment of a bay and tidelands at Pt. Mugu, California. At that time, he was seventy-five years old and his only fault was that he kept leaving people forty years his junior behind as he walked in the mud flats and tidal areas.

"His wife, Nettie, was only sixty-five years old so we made no attempt to keep up with her when the going was heavy. One day, the "young" folks of thirty to forty-five years were asking the MacGinities how they were able to be so active with no signs of arthritis, back trouble, or other bone problems.

The MacGinities told them that they had taken a tablespoon of sea water on their cereal every day for forty years, and when they were away from the ocean, they used sea salt instead of salt mined from the land. Sea salt is made by evaporating sea water in large ponds using the sun's rays. They did not say that their robust good health was only because of using sea water or salt, but their explanation for using the sea source was because there might be something missing in land-mined salt."

The formula for sea water-reinforced distilled water is as follows: Add four teaspoons of unheated, filtered sea water to one-half gallon of distilled water. Refrigerate.

If you wish to use sea salt, use the following formula: To one pint of distilled water, add one-eighth (⅛) teaspoon of ground *whole* sea salt. (This whole sea salt, which includes *all* minerals in balance, comes from France or Belgium and is found in health food stores.)

It is my sincere hope that every distilling manufac-

45

turer will circulate these formulas to everyone who uses a distiller, to avoid mineral loss in the body and avoid the risk of health problems caused by this loss.

References

1. George L. Waldbott. *A Struggle with Titans.* New York, N.Y.: Carlton Press, 1965.
2. *Archives of Pathology.* vol. 73, no. 5, May 1962.
3. *Consumer Bulletin.* March 1973.
4. *New England Journal of Medicine.* no. 280, pp. 805-807, 1969.
5. Ruth Adams and Frank Murray. *Minerals: Kill or Cure?* New York, N.Y.: Larchmont Books, 1974.
6. *Organic Consumer Report.* vol. 52, no. 15, 11 April 1972.
7. Ibid.

You Can See
the Difference

Is THERE really a difference between natural and synthetic vitamins and minerals? Some supplement companies produce products from natural sources exclusively. Others make them from synthetics only. Still others combine both. Are all products the same in effect? What is the truth?

Most scientists claim that natural and synthetic vitamins and minerals are identical. Why do they believe this? How is a vitamin synthesized? Why is it synthesized?

The method of synthesis, generally speaking, is this: A single vitamin factor, called a crystalline substance, is separated from its natural source, such as rice polishings, brewer's yeast, liver, citrus fruits, etc. It then becomes an isolated factor. Once it is isolated, its molecular formation or pattern is determined; then it is duplicated in the chemical laboratory by assembling component parts from chemicals already available. Some of these chemicals are coal-tar products. The synthetic vitamins are then presumably identical to the natural crystalline vitamins which they imitate. They have the same molecular formations and the same chemical reactions, according to chemists who insist that no one can tell the difference.

Why are vitamins synthesized? Because synthetics are cheaper to produce than the natural.

However, though the isolated factor may appear identical, there is one undisputed difference between a natural and a synthetic product. Natural vitamins are derived or condensed from natural foods. In these natural foods many factors occur together: vitamins, minerals, amino acids and enzymes, which help the body utilize absorbable nutrients. Researchers are learning that *all of these factors work as a team*. When one is separated or torn away from the companions with which it grew, the natural balance is disturbed.

Nutrition research is finding that when these associated factors—known or unknown—are separated or removed, their utilization within the body is often disturbed. There are hundreds of examples already known, and more are being discovered as time passes. For example, it is already well known that vitamin D is needed for the assimilation of calcium. Calcium and phosphorus work as a team. Vitamin A is now reported to enhance the assimilation of vitamin E. Vitamin K has recently been found to protect against a deficiency of vitamin C. Usually these factors occur together in nature.

John J. Miller, Ph.D., a biochemist who has spent a lifetime studying these interrelationships, believes that man has not identified all the nutrients—nor the necessary interrelationships between the nutrients—let alone learned how to apply them to health. He says that man does not know all the elements which exist in plants and natural foods, nor how these nutrients are combined into a balance of vitamins, minerals, amino acids (protein factors) and enzymes.

Dr. Miller states, "We simply do not know enough . . . [to] ever be able to improve on Nature's plan of enzyme interrelationships."

Is this proof that natural vitamins are better?

The late Eugene Schiff explained it this way: "I believe it is wrong to say natural vitamins are better. In their crystalline or isolated form they may not be. The right way to say it is that natural vitamin *preparations* made from the whole foods or food concentrates are better to the extent that they contain other factors besides the individual vitamin. ...

"If we want, for instance, one milligram of natural vitamin B-1 or thiamin, we do not put into a tablet one milligram of natural vitamin B-1, but 200 milligrams of yeast. The real difference in what the user gets is the other 199 milligrams present in the yeast, the associated factors which obviously cannot be present in one milligram of straight or synthetic B-1."

How can you tell whether a preparation is natural? Labels may give a clue. For example, to determine whether vitamin E is from synthetic or natural sources, the vitamin E can be examined in the laboratory by a chemical process. In natural vitamin E the molecules rotate light to the right, called dextro-rotatory or abbreviated as *d*. Synthetic E, examined by this same laboratory process, reveals equal portions of right and left molecules, designated by the letters *dl*. The average buyer cannot make this test himself, so he must search the labels, which unfortunately change from time to time. However, any vitamin E preparations marketed today are natural if they have the following labels*:

d-alpha tocopherol
d-alpha tocopheryl acetate
d-alpha tocopheryl succinate
mixed tocopherols

Synthetic vitamin E preparations which are marketed today will be labeled as follows:

dl-alpha tocopherol
dl-alpha tocopheryl acetate
dl-alpha tocopheryl succinate [from Europe]

---

*Courtesy of J. R. Carlson Laboratories, Inc., Chicago, which specialize in natural vitamin E.

Buy other vitamins from a reputable firm specializing in natural vitamins.

Does this mean that you should avoid synthetic vitamins completely? Not necessarily. Studies show that certain fish cannot live in synthetic or artificial sea water, but when some natural sea water is added to the artificial, they can exist. Studies also show that certain isolated synthetic vitamins accomplish specific actions, i.e., nudging a sluggish or deficient cell or organ or tissue back into working order. However, many nutritional physicians feel that administration of these synthetic vitamins in massive amounts should be medically supervised. The reason: After the necessary stimulation has been achieved (nutritional physicians can determine this), the large amounts of synthetics become similar in action to drugs. Their continued administration is like whipping a tired horse. At that point, nutritional physicians believe, natural vitamin *preparations*, complete with *all* nutrients, known and unknown, should be used as maintenance therapy. They consider them safer in the long run. But there is another reason.

All due credit should go to the chemists who have isolated and synthesized vitamin factors. They have proved helpful in certain circumstances, as just described. But Rudolph Hauschka, D.Sc., has been at work for decades on laboratory experiments which show the dissimilarity between natural and synthetic vitamins and the difference in their effect. He explains how we learned about vitamins in the first place. In 1882 one group of animals was fed synthetic milk, while another group was given natural milk. The animals fed fresh milk grew up to be lively; those on synthetic milk died. The logical conclusion was that there must be "something" in natural milk which had escaped chemical detection, but was important to life. This hypothetical substance was later (in 1912) called a "vitamin." This led to a tidal wave of research and the discovery of many vitamins. However, nutrition is in its infancy. We still have not discovered all the factors in food. Twenty years ago vitamin B-12 was thought to be the final discovery in the B complex. Today we know there is a vitamin B-22, and there are no doubt more to come.

An experiment in Dr. Hauschka's laboratory ascertained that single synthetic substances were indistinguishable from the natural, according to available tests, but it was found that there was a difference in *effect*. The doctor learned that synthetics of coal-tar origin are effective *only in allopathic dosage* (i.e., usual drug dosages), *but in homeopathic dilutions they are useless*. He says, "Thus it is fair to say that a basic biological difference exists between natural and synthetic products, despite their chemical identity. Laboratory experiments prove this (1)."

Now for a surprise. Other scientists have found a way to distinguish a natural vitamin formula from a synthetic. The sensitive crystallizations of natural nutrients *can be photographed*. The results, called "chromatograms," look a little like snowflakes but are in color. An analysis of foods, or natural substances, by these chromatograms will show a definite pattern, whereas the synthetics will not have a pattern. The natural patterns can be translated into vitamin and mineral organizations. Those which have no pattern are considered by the researchers who discovered this process to be non-nutritious and valueless as foods.

Dr. Gerhard Schmidt of Switzerland, a follower of Rudolf Steiner, has long worked in this field. He has photographed chromatograms which reveal the differences between soils treated with chemical fertilizers and those treated with natural fertilizers. The difference, as proved by the chromatograms, is also visible in the foods grown on these soils (i.e., the chromatogram of an organically grown carrot differs from one grown as usual). Chromatograms also show the effect processing has on natural foods. For example, a chromatogram shows that strength is taken away from rice when it is "peeled" and polished. And flour which is stone-ground appears different from that produced by the commercial milling process which removes many natural factors (2).

This is truly exciting news!

Actually, this method of photographing the crystalline structure in food elements is not new. About 1903, a Dr. Abbott in Australia was the first to experiment with the idea, using osmosis. Later, around 1926, the Doctors Kolisko, a man-and-wife M.D. team, improved upon the Abbott process, combining osmosis with metalized crystallization. They called this method "Capillary Dynamolytical Testing." These two doctors devoted their lives to this subject and made millions of experiments on natural foods. Their rare book, now out of print but soon to be reprinted, is called, *Agriculture of Tomorrow.*

The late Dr. Ehrenfried Pfeiffer, of the Biochemical Research Laboratories in this country, considered by many chemists as the greatest biochemist of our time, was a student of the Koliskos and brought the dynamolytical testing method to this country from England. Dr. Pfeiffer also photographed many chromatograms in his laboratory.

He stated, "Various undulations and spike formations in a pattern enable researchers to recognize biological activity and intrinsic values not revealed in highly refined or synthetic preparations."

References

1. Rudolph Hauschka, D.Sc. *The Nature of Substance.* London: Vincent Stuart Ltd., 1966. (German text, 1950.)
2. Dr. G. Schmidt. *Beitrage.* No. 24, 1966, through No. 29, 1968; Dornach, Switzerland.

For Women Only

A GROUP of us was discussing nutrition in a business meeting. I commented that for some unexplainable reason, I had received a deluge of questions concerning women's ailments, all within one week's time. A health store had called to ask me to write an article because so many customers needed help. A friend, a father of several daughters, called long distance pleading for information. He said he was tired of listening to the moaning and groaning of his daughters with "female complaints." I even had a letter from India from an American university graduate who was seeking knowledge of what foods and vitamins would help her through menopause—all in the same week!

One man in the group to whom I was making these comments looked surprised and said, "You mean that *nutrition* can improve or reverse the side effects of menstruation and menopause?" He looked incredulous.

"Of course," I answered.

Later, after the meeting broke up, this man drew up a chair and said, "For goodness' sake, tell me about it." I judged by the expression on his face and the tone of his voice that he, as well as a wife, daughter or a sister, were victims of the miseries that often accompany women's ailments, and that can be upsetting to the entire family.

After reminding him that I am a nutrition reporter who searches for the findings of various experts in the field and do not prescribe, I began to tell him what many of these experts had learned about the effects of nutrition on such disturbances.

"Many women are said to become 'witches' during the premenstrual period," I told him. "Adelle Davis told of a woman who said, 'That's the time I spank the kids, yell at my husband, live on tranquilizers and can't stand myself' (1).

"Another investigator," I continued, "is Dr. Erle Henriksen, of the University of California, who conducted a three-year study of 200 women. He said: 'It takes extremely stable husbands and children to put up with the worst sufferers. Some husbands just run and hide. Others ask for divorce. It's a very serious problem and completely unnecessary because it can be prevented'" (2).

My friend looked as if he had already experienced the entire problem. He asked, "What causes such a change of personality in an otherwise sweet and intelligent woman?"

I answered, "Of course, these emotional problems can occur at any age—in teenagers, middle-aged women and later during menopause. However one cause, according to investigators, is the same: lack of calcium. About a week or ten days prior to menstruation, the blood calcium begins to drop. This drop in what might be called the 'nerve mineral' can produce all sorts of nervous complaints: insomnia, irritability, tension, quick anger, quarrelsomeness, depression, anxiety, headaches—the works. Adolescents as well as older women may burst into tears at the slightest provocation. Then when menstruation actually begins, the calcium in the blood drops still further. This can cause cramps and if the calcium deficiency is severe, even convulsions may occur. Apparently there is also a relationship between calcium and the production of hormones."

"Will taking calcium prevent these disturbances?" the man asked. "If so, how much?"

"Adelle Davis stated that both premenstrual tension as well as cramps can be prevented if calcium is begun about ten days prior to menstruation and continued through the second or third day. In case of cramps, she suggested taking one or two calcium tablets every hour. Nutritionists consider calcium a natural tranquilizer and far safer than drugs (3).

"That isn't the whole story," I added hastily because my friend looked as if he were anxious to rush home immediately and start administering calcium to the female department of his family. "In addition, blood sugar drops, and with it energy. Women often crave sweets as a result, and become thirsty. Then they begin to store water. Abdomens bloat, breasts swell and become sensitive, and weight increases much to the disgust of the victim. Fortunately, though, there is new help for this problem."

My listener grabbed an old envelope out of his pocket and began to scribble notes furiously.

"John M. Ellis, M.D., of Texas," I continued, "has done considerable research with vitamin B-6 on women who store water during pregnancy, premenstrual periods or menopause, and found that as long as they took vitamin B-6 daily, they were no longer bothered with this problem. But when the B-6 was stopped, the results ceased. Dr. Ellis's explanation is that apparently B-6 sets up a balance between two minerals, sodium and potassium, which in turn regulate the body fluids (4).

"But what is even more exciting, the good results were not limited to women. Cattlemen who rode the vast Texas ranges, and had complained of tingling and numbness of fingers and toes as well as excruciating night cramps in the calves of their legs, were relieved of these symptoms within a few weeks by B-6. Best of all, without cutting calories, these men lost weight because of the loss of fluid in their bodies."

"How much B-6 did Dr. Ellis give his patients?" my listener asked.

"He gave them 50 mg daily in most cases and said that after three years of this daily dosage there were no side effects. However, those who work in nutrition believe that it is always wise to take the entire B complex along with large amounts of a single B vitamin. Otherwise too much of one has been known to create a deficiency of another. Anyway, since vitamin B also helps nerves, in addition to calcium, this is all to the good."

"You didn't say what to do about the low blood sugar problem," he reminded me.

"That isn't hard," I answered. "Avoid sugar and other carbohydrates, and cut down on coffee, all of which cause a temporary rise of blood sugar and energy followed by a nose dive of both. Substitute fresh fruit to satisfy a craving for sweets, and use protein instead of carbohydrates. Nuts, or cheese or stirring some brewer's yeast (high in protein) into juice or water and drinking it together with taking a calcium tablet or so, has been known to change irritable teenagers or wives into veritable angels temporarily and quickly. The energy appears within about ten minutes and can last several hours.

"If a person suffers continuously from low blood sugar (hypoglycemia) not only at premenstrual times, she would be wise to consult an M.D. who specializes in hypoglycemia.

"The last is the best of all," I said. "It is true that hormones are involved in all of these women's ailments. Sometimes there are too many, sometimes there are not enough. There is a vitamin, sometimes loosely called the 'sex vitamin,' which appears to act as a natural hormone regulator. It is vitamin E. If a woman has lived through premenstrual tension, she can live through menopause, but believe me it will be much easier if she has vitamin E to help her. I can cite the testimonies of scores of friends and relatives. The only symptoms which differ between menstruation and menopause are hot flashes, peculiar to menopause, and sometimes scanty or excessive blood flow. Just listen to what vitamin E has accomplished for menopause sufferers:

"Dr. N. R. Kavinoky reported that from 10 to 25 units daily of vitamin E gave 37 out of 92 patients relief from hot flashes; 16 relief from backache; 34 relief from excessive menstrual flow. Dr. C. J. Christy found that 10 to 30 units of vitamin E daily brought such great improvement to menopausal patients that they lost their dread of menopause. Dr. Henry Gozan reported that he used a much higher dosage. He treated 35 menopausal patients with 300 units of vitamin E daily, in conjunction with good nutrition. Nineteen were improved or completely relieved within two to four weeks (5). Friends of mine who tried vitamin E decided, when their hot flashes improved, that it was 'all in their mind' or the flashes would have stopped anyway, and gave up the vitamin E. They changed their tune in a hurry when the flashes returned with a vengeance until they resumed the vitamin."

"Is there any danger of taking too much vitamin E?" my friend asked.

"Yes," I answered. "In cases of high blood pressure, where it should be started very gradually, or in people with rheumatic fever, caution should be observed, according to Wilfrid E. Shute, M.D. His book suggests dosages (6).

"E. V. Shute, M.D., his brother and co-worker in vitamin E therapy, says, 'Certainly there are no people who cannot take 50 units of vitamin E safely. There are virtually no people who cannot take 100 units safely, unless allergy exists. . . . Now with increasing deficiency [it is often removed from our food] it may take a large dose to prevent trouble' (7).

"Dr. Wilfrid Shute also warns that vitamin E should not be given at the same time as inorganic iron (derived from chemical, not from food sources) or with the female hormone, estrogen, since both of these substances cancel out vitamin E. They should be taken twelve hours apart, i.e., one in the morning, and the other[s] in the evening" (8).

"I am glad you mentioned estrogen," my listener said. "There is so much controversy about female hormones; should women take them or not?"

"Apparently one should not generalize," I answered. "Individuals differ. Dr. Melvin Page, of the Page Biochemical Foundation, once told me that some women do not manufacture enough estrogen, while others do manufacture enough. He believed, as a result of thousands of patients and detailed blood chemistry tests, that it was safe to give estrogen to women who *under* secreted it. He did not believe it was safe to give it to those who secreted it sufficiently. Of course, during menopause, when hormonal output is slowing down, it may be necessary, but results should be watched carefully by a physician.

"In some menopausal women there is 'flooding.' If vitamin E does not control this situation, a physician may resort to estrogen. Alan H. Nittler, M.D. says, 'The female hormone tablets can be of great value during menopause. Estrogens are supplied in two forms: synthetic and natural. The synthetic is more powerful and the natural less likely to lead to malignancy. Of course the dosage is an individual thing.' "

"How is it given?" my friend asked.

"Dr. Page always has given it orally in 1/1000 of the

usual pharmaceutical dosage," I answered. "He feels that this tiny amount, like homeopathic potencies, does a better job than massive doses. Dr. Nittler often gives it by injection. However, he points out that in some women this may *cause* a hemorrhage. If so, he substitutes wheat germ oil by mouth. He explains, 'I use a product which is an 8:1 concentration of wheat germ oil. This preparation contains some of the natural precursors to the sex hormone. If taken over a long enough time and in adequate amounts, it should bring the desired results. Sometimes as many as thirty tablets a day are necessary to control excessive bleeding. Vitamin K may also be indicated.'

"One final tip for excessive bleeders comes from Carlton Fredricks, Ph.D. He points out that in young people, particularly, there may be an excess of female hormones. It is the job of the liver to detoxify these excess hormones. The liver cannot do this job properly if it is congested with carbohydrates, toxins, chemicals and drugs or insecticides. (Dr. Kurt W. Donsbach has an excellent and easy liver-detoxifying plan (9).) And to avoid the pooped out feeling as a result of excessive bleeding, most doctors prescribe iron and/or vitamin B-12."

My friend pushed back his chair as he realized I had finished and said, "I wish I had known all this long ago."

"Well," I said, "it's never too late to begin except that it may take longer to correct long-term deficiencies. However, according to these researchers I have mentioned, you now have a kit of tools to apply to ailments of any woman in your family: calcium, vitamin B-6 (plus the whole B complex), protein, vitamin E and of course a nutritionally rich diet. Nature did not intend that women should suffer from these ailments which are part of the life process. As proof, primitive women, living on a whole, natural, primitive diet did not have them. They returned to work in the fields almost immediately after giving birth to a child. Perhaps it is time to get closer to nature. At any rate, many women who have used these natural nutritional substances will testify that their ailments have definitely improved."

References

1. Adelle Davis. *Let's Get Well.* New York, N.Y.: Harcourt Brace Jovanovich, 1965.
2. Linda Clark. *Stay Young Longer.* New York, N.Y.: Pyramid Publications, 1968.
3. *Let's Get Well.*
4. John Ellis, M.D. *The Doctor Who Looked at Hands.* New York, N.Y.: Arco Books, 1970.
5. *Stay Young Longer.*
6. Wilfrid E. Shute, M.D. *Dr. Wilfrid E. Shute's Complete, Updated Vitamin E Book.* New Canaan, Conn.: Keats Publishing, 1975.
7. *Stay Young Longer.*
8. *Dr. Shute's Complete, Updated Vitamin E Book.*
9. Dr. Kurt W. Donsbach. *Preventive Organic Medicine.* New Canaan, Conn.: Keats Publishing, 1976.

Poking Holes in
Some Old Theories
on Nutrition

FOR A LONG TIME, nutritionists laid down certain basic
rules for everyone. One rule concerned fixed amounts of
vitamins that everyone is supposed to need. Another was
that everyone, no exceptions allowed, should eat a big
breakfast, a light lunch, and a still lighter dinner. This
plan sounded sensible when it was explained that the
greater amount of fuel is needed during the earlier part
of the day, when activity is greater, and less at the end
of the day when it isn't. Those who complained (and I
was among them) that they weren't hungry enough to
eat a big breakfast were told that the real trouble was, if
you eat a big dinner at night you aren't hungry enough
to cope with a big breakfast. Still another rule (and as a
nutrition reporter I, too, have dutifully passed it on to
the readers) was that everyone needs a high protein,
moderate fat, and low carbohydrate diet. Now, according to some recent discoveries, the old, established rules
have been found not to work *for some people*.

With all due respect to the nutritionists, such hard
and fast rules may indeed apply only to the average person. But we are beginning to learn that average or "normal" are unreliable designations. Roger J. Williams,
Ph.D., was the first to shoot holes in the theory that we
are all alike and thus need the same amount of vitamins.
He learned this through extensive laboratory tests with

animals and people. Each of us is as different as our fingerprints. Antomy textbooks show pictures proving that our hearts and other organs vary in size, our digestions differ and our needs for certain amounts of vitamins differ accordingly. So there went one rule down the drain.

Now comes another researcher, George Watson, Ph.D., who insists that big breakfasts are not wise for all people and the same amount of protein isn't either. This announcement made me sit bolt upright with surprise. For years I have been trying to make myself eat big breakfasts because I thought I should. Yet my husband could hardly wait until breakfast, at which time he ate with gusto fruit, steak, hashed brown potatoes, toasted English muffins and liberal amounts of coffee. As he patted his stomach complacently afterwards, he would say with strong conviction: "Everybody should eat a big breakfast like that." But so help me, I couldn't! The very thought of such a big meal first thing in the morning, regardless of the size of my previous night's dinner, was too much for me to face. Yet by dinner time I welcomed the idea most heartily while my husband ordered soup.

Recently, a friend wrote me about a new book which challenges some of these ironclad nutritional rules. She said· "At long last, someone agrees with me. I *hate* big breakfasts and I have never thrived on them. Now there is a researcher with information that *some people* should not eat them."

I promptly bought George Watson's book, *Nutrition and Your Mind* (1). Dr. Watson is a biopsychologist and psychochemist who taught mathematical logic and philosophy of science at USC, before settling down to work with doctors and psychiatrists on full-time research in psychochemistry, which means the use of certain nutrients for the mentally and emotionally disturbed.

As for physical differences, Dr. Watson found that people react differently to different methods of eating as well as to different foods; an idea we all should have suspected long ago. Dr. Watson believes, as a result of some twenty years of study, that there are two main types of eaters—the fast oxidizers and the slow oxidizers. (The term *oxidizer* means the speed with which the body breaks down food to be used for energy.) Each type, he says, can thrive on or suffer from eating certain foods which produce just the opposite results in the other type. He provides a questionnaire in his book to help you decide which type you are. I will outline the rudiments of each type to give you some idea of the differences between them. However, Dr. Watson makes it clear that these two types may not be "normal." In fact, he states that the body chemistry of each is out of kilter, and he is hopeful that certain nutrients will help to establish at least near-normalcy. Not everyone will agree with everything Dr. Watson says, and in the years to come, he may disagree with himself on some of the points.

Nevertheless, Dr. Watson stretches our thinking. The questionnaire results are not even absolute. Several people have told me that their answer was not an either/or, but both/and. In other words, some people have some characteristics of both fast and slow oxidizers, but may have a stronger leaning toward one than the other. At any rate, it is fun to get a general idea of your tendencies. There are some startling ideas to consider which may do us all some good. Meanwhile use a grain of salt in choosing your type.

The Fast Oxidizer

- Burns too much sugar
- Does not break down sufficient amounts of fats and protein

- Apparently thrives on big breakfasts
- Hates coffee and gets an unpleasant reaction from it
- Prefers tea without lemon
- Finds grapefruit and other sour foods too sharp for his tastes
- May be upset by raw onions, green peppers
- Usually becomes weak if he goes two or three hours without eating
- Feels better on a low carbohydrate, high fat, high protein diet
- Gets relief from antacids; is more prone to acid stomach
- Is more sensitive, emotional, and likely to take offense quickly

The Slow Oxidizer

- Burns too little sugar
- Eats too much protein and fat
- Doesn't like big breakfasts nor feel good after them
- Likes somewhat weak coffee, which speeds him up a bit (but one shouldn't become dependent on it)
- Likes sour things, such as vinegar, pickles, lemonade and tea with lemon
- Loves raw onions, green peppers
- Can go hours without eating, perhaps with only one (evening) meal
- Feels better on a high carbohydrate, low fat, low protein diet
- Is the more placid type

Dr. Watson believes that even though these two types of eaters are not physically or nutritionally normal, if a person does not feel well or becomes depressed on his

present diet, he might feel better by changing his diet to
fit his type.

Here are the general classifications of foods Dr. Watson suggests for each:

Fast Oxidizers

- Should avoid sweets except those high in fat, low
  in flour. But they may eat the following:
- Vegetables: avocados, artichoke hearts, peas,
  beans, lentils, cauliflower, spinach and asparagus
- Proteins: Organ meats (liver, kidneys, etc.),
  sardines, caviar, anchovies, herring, meat gravies
- Fats: butter

Slow Oxidizers

- May eat more sweets and starches such as potatoes, rice, bread and cereals. They may eat the
  following:
- Salads: lettuce, green peppers, onions, radishes,
  cabbage, pickles, cucumbers
- Proteins: milk, buttermilk, [yogurt], cottage
  cheese, eggs, fish, but not the proteins recommended for fast oxidizers
- Regular coffee (in moderation), catsup, spicy
  sauces

Unfortunately, Dr. Watson does not make a distinc-
tion between natural and processed sweets, foods and
beverages, so nutritionists are not going to take all of his
food suggestions lying down—as they shouldn't. His re-
marks about alcohol *are* supported by other researchers,
however: "If you think you need a drink, you don't;
you need nourishment, instead. And if you can hold
your liquor, there is something wrong with your body. A
truly healthy person cannot tolerate alcohol."

Dr. Watson does admit that food—right or wrong—is
not the only cause of poor health or even of depression.

Sulfa drugs, poisons such as napthalene (found in moth-balls or crystals), ammonia, pesticides, as well as fumes of drying paint, have caused such troubles as depression, nausea and loss of appetite in sensitive people.

Dr. Watson recommends the following vitamins and minerals as being especially helpful for each type:

Fast Oxidizers

- A, E
- B-12, B-3 (niacin), pantothenic acid, choline, inositol—(all are B vitamins)
- C—both ascorbic acid and the bioflavonoids
- Minerals: calcium, phosphorus, iodine, zinc sul-fate

Slow Oxidizers

- B-1, B-2, B-6, PABA, niacin
- Ascorbic acid (C)
- D
- Minerals: potassium, magnesium, copper, man-ganese, iron

Unfortunately, again, the vitamins and minerals Dr. Watson advocates are synthetic as well as incomplete, and one iron product he recommends in his book has actually been found dangerous. (After all, one cannot be an expert in everything and Dr. Watson obviously is not a vitamin-mineral researcher per se.)

Dr. Watson limits his vitamins. Dr. Roger J. Williams, the developer of one vitamin and a pioneer in the use of another, states emphatically that the body needs *all* vitamins and minerals as well as optimum nutrition to build and maintain health, even though the amounts may vary from person to person, according to the needs of each. Dr. Williams has proved this in laboratory experiments and is honored the world over for his discoveries.

Actually, whatever your type seems to be, *you* are the only one to know what food does or does not agree with you. The only traps involving this "wisdom of the body" are the false appetites or cravings for sugar, alcohol, coffee and tobacco. For most people, these are habit-forming and the more one has, the more one wants. These cravings cannot be trusted.

One observation about the desires of the fast vs. the slow oxidizers concerns the aversion to, or craving for, sour things. Usually the craving is a sign that the body is crying for more hydrochloric acid, and if it is taken, the slow oxidizer could assimilate more protein as well as minerals, both of which require HCl for complete digestion. Remember that Dr. Watson does consider these two types of eaters abnormal, and each type of blood chemistry out of kilter. But recognition of the difference may spur people toward optimum nutrition which may help correct the sharper differences, at least. For example, a friend, who through the Watson questionnaire learned she was a slow oxidizer, immediately began to improve her overall nutrition. She feels definitely better and believes that a six-month re-check will find her with more normal responses.

Dr. Watson may not yet have all the answers and much more research is obviously needed. However, I truly believe he has discovered something others have overlooked: that people do indeed vary according to food preferences and assimilation. This may also be a factor in reducing. It may explain why that size eight wife could eat more than her large husband. One may be a fast oxidizer, the other a slow oxidizer.

This clarification may be a new breakthrough in nutrition which will be enlightening to many people. At least, I am no longer going to feel guilty when I refuse to eat a big breakfast!

References

1. George Watson, Ph.D. *Nutrition and Your Mind.* Los Angeles, Cal.: Phoenix House, 1974.

The Truth about Breakfast Cereals

IN 1970 another bombshell dropped on the American scene of health and nutrition—the exposé of dry, processed cereals. Although this information no doubt amazed the general public who have long been consuming these cereals—as well as forcing them down the throats of their children—it was no surprise to those who already knew the truth.

The bombshell came from a painstakingly compiled report by Robert B. Choate, a former nutrition consultant to Presidential adviser Dr. Jean Mayer, and presented to the Senate Consumer Subcommittee.

As columnist Jack Anderson wrote: "The evidence shows all six of the big breakfast-food giants are guilty of phony advertising."

Choate pointed out that the heavily advertised dry cereals actually contain only "empty" calories; that they can keep people fat but not necessarily healthy; that presweetened cereals may lead to consumption of too much sugar; and that actually the main source of nutrition of these cereals is the added milk and fruit served with them. In fact, he said, "Some of the most heavily advertised cereals have about as much nutritional value as a shot of whiskey. They fatten but do little to prevent malnutrition."

Choate, who was armed with charts, graphs and samples of television ads, told the Senate subcommittee:

"It is apparent . . . we humans are viewed not so much as beings to be nourished as suckers to be sold."

Did the breakfast food companies take this adverse publicity lying down? Of course not. They are still screaming, "Lies! Lies!" and recruiting all the rooters for their side they can get from "leading nutritional authorities in the nation who do not agree with Mr. Choate" and "experts in the field, the medical profession and dietitians" to convince the public to the contrary.

Well, what is the truth? The late Fred D. Miller, a dentist from Altoona, Pennsylvania, author of *Open Door to Health, A Proven Program for Dental and Physical Health through Proper Nutrition*, stated that while he was attending a Midwest dental society meeting he decided to visit one of the most famous breakfast food factories. "I wanted to see with my own eyes how breakfast food manufacturers treated corn and rice as well as wheat in making breakfast foods," he said.

"First I saw machinery removing the outer coat, then the germ (in other words, the life) from corn. This, my guide explained, was to prevent their cornflakes from 'rancidity and spoilage' . . . What was left of the corn at this point had an unlifelike pallor as befits any corpse. Masses of this corpse-like substance (I refuse to call it corn) were put in large pressure cookers heated to a temperature of 250 degrees and held at that temperature for two-and-a-half hours, when it was ready to be mixed with artificial flavoring and coloring to make it look and taste less the corpse it really was.

"The entire mass was then cooled until it reached a stage at which it was ready to be run through machines to flake it. At this point it began a journey on endless belts that passed it through heaters where it reached a temperature of 450 degrees, thus assuring loss or deterioration of nutritional elements that might have survived up to then. The process 'set' the flakes to prevent them from sticking together. Now it was ready for packaging in cartons lined with waxed paper. This, said the guide, would keep their product 'as fresh as a daisy.' The factory was sending out sixty-five carloads of this foodless pap and other breakfast foods to be eaten by human beings. . . . In my estimation, if you eat the label, the carton and its waxed-paper lining you get just about as much live food value as when you eat what is inside. Since my visit another process has been added: the insertion of synthetic vitamins" (1).

Adelle Davis added: " 'Enriched' cereals, like 'enriched' flour have been robbed of some twenty nutrients; little worth mentioning is put back. Most packaged cereals have been far more successful as money makers than as health builders" (2).

When W. H. Sebrell, M.D., was serving with the United States Public Health Service, he said: "To me it does seem a little ridiculous to take a natural foodstuff in which the vitamins and minerals have been placed by nature, submit this foodstuff to a refining process which removes them, and then add them back to the refined product at an increased cost" (3).

As if that were not enough, something still newer has been added. Just try and find a dry cereal in a supermarket that is not embellished with the highly suspect "freshness preservers," BHT and BHA, topped off with a long list of other chemicals.

BHA and BHT are not limited to cereals but are added to nearly every packaged food to increase shelf life. Recently I was in a grocery store which sells both regular and gourmet foods. I was searching the cracker department for some whole wheat crackers fit to eat, when another customer joined me and asked me if I knew about those "delicious, crispy, whole wheat crackers which crinkle at the edges." I had never heard of them, so she asked the store owner who promptly produced a big box of them. The woman fell upon them with glee and tore open the box to offer me one. I ate it and it *was* delicious. The woman said, "Now *you* buy a box!"

I answered, "Not until I read the label." I scrutinized it, and there, not to my surprise, BHA and BHT were listed. I said, "No, I cannot buy these; they contain BHA and BHT. I will not risk it." She looked at me suspiciously and asked what BHA and BHT were. I said, "They are preservatives, and as a starter, when fed to rats they cause the baby rats to be born blind."

The woman looked daggers at me and said, "This is just the reason I refuse to read labels," and she stamped out of the store so fast and furiously, she forgot to pay for the box of crackers.

This is what I call hiding your head in the sand like an ostrich. If customers *would* read labels and complain, the manufacturers would act. Preservatives have already been removed from one cereal due to consumer complaints. But we need more complaints against other nonnutritive foods or those which have been overloaded with additives to help the manufacturer, not the consumer.

What About Effect on Health?

Dr. Ralph Bircher, of the famous nutritional Bircher-Benner Clinic in Switzerland, says: "The regular consumption of devitalized food which has been overprocessed (and is thus far from its natural state) . . . may impair health. . . . A healthy organism can deal with these foods as an occasional exception but not if they become a daily habit" (4).

After learning about the ruthless refining of dry cereals, Dr. Miller forbade his patients to touch them. He discovered that substituting natural whole foods produced not only excellent teeth and gums, but good health, vigor, and mental alertness. (His book describes his nutritional program.) Many of his dental patients came to him as tiny children and remained under his care as adults. One is a movie star with radiant health as well as beautiful teeth. Two other patients made headlines—two little boys who were started and maintained on this natural whole food regime. When they reached their teens, they were chosen for a university study of a large group of Pennsylvania school children and tested in eight different medical-nutritional examinations. *Of 2,536 students they were found to have perfect teeth and were rated BEST in all eight health tests*! This, in spite of the fact that their four grandparents were wearing full sets of dentures in their toothless jaws (5).

What Cereals Are Best?

Even though the original bombshell against presweetened packaged cereals was dropped in 1970, as late as October, 1974, few reforms had taken place. TV commercials were still luring children to eat them, and the sugar industry was still insisting that sugar is an "energy food," which many people still believe. Yet truly dedicated natural food converts avoid adding sugar to anything. They may use a bit of honey, or fresh fruit, but sugar? No! Why?

Sugar has been found to cause a variety of disturbances including obesity, dental decay, heart disease, diabetes and hypoglycemia. Dr. John Yudkin, of England, discovered the connection between sugar and heart disease; some Israeli citizens living on a low sugar diet were found to have less diabetes than others, living in the same country, who ate more sweets; dental decay in 225 Swedish children was lowered 30 percent when they substituted sugarless snacks, according to a study at the Stockholm Dental School (6).

Yet the promotion of presweetened cereals continues unabated. Dr. Jean Mayer states, "The promotion of high-sugar cereals, snacks and soft drinks to children is a dental disaster, and may be a factor in increasing the likelihood of diabetes in generically vulnerable subjects. For the past two years consumption of sugar and corn syrup has exceeded our flour consumption with unpredictable results for the health of the country" (7).

The Center for Science in the Public Interest, a public service group in Washington, D.C., has petitioned the Food and Drug Administration to attach a warning label to all cereals containing more than 10 percent sugar. Since the manufacturers are loathe to disclose the amount in their cereals, Dr. Michael Jacobson, co-director of the public service group, calculated the sugar content of some of the major brands. The findings, in percentages, are as follows:

King Vitamins	50	Cocoa Pebbles	44
Fruity Pebbles	44	Super Sugar Crisp	43
Sir Grapefellow	40	Post Alpha-Bits	40
Cocoa Crispies	38	Captain Crunch	37
Fruit Loops	35	Super Sugar Corn Chex	33
Sugar Frosted Flakes	29	Mr. Wonderful Surprise	29
Post Oak Flakes	20	100% Natural	19
Corn Chex	14	Life	14
Product 19	12	Total	11
Concentrate	11	Wheaties	11
Special K	9	Corn Flakes	7
Rice Krispies	7	Post Toasties	7
Raisin Bran	6	Wheat Chex	6
Rice Chex	5	Cheerios	4

But the cereal manufacturers are still in there pitching. The director of public affairs for the Kellogg Company, an estimated $800 million-a-year cereal industry, stated, "It is outrageous that fear-mongering consumerists continue to slander the food industry, libel the Kellogg Company, and frighten America's parents."

The president of the Cereal Institute is even more tear-jerking in his statement: "To force presweetened cereals off the market would deprive children of the nutrients they now obtain in a form they find attractive, and could result in a deterioration of their health" (8).

Healthful nutrients in those cereals? Listen to what Adelle Davis said about them. "A university took the 'ten best' advertised cereals, those directed to children and promising to 'build champions,' mixed them together and fed them to rats. Within six weeks all the rats died. Then the cereal manufacturers complained that their cereals were not eaten alone, but with milk and fruit. So the university researchers ground up the empty cardboard boxes of the 'ten best,' added milk and fruit, and fed the mixture to the animals. The rats thrived!" (9).

Although Mr. Choate's list of cereals rated three at the top and five as "nutritionally meritorious," in our opinion he did not have much choice in the category which he studied. Those with higher nutritional ratings are still synthetically "enriched." Our approach would be to choose cereals of a different kind altogether. There is a wonderful selection of both cold and hot cereals, if you know what to look for and where to get them. They are delicious as well as nutritious. They can also be health builders and come closer to making good the empty promises made for the commercial dry cereals.

Steel-cut oats (not subjected to the heat of rollers, which diminishes nutrients), cooked or uncooked, are one choice. Gaylord Hauser, in his cookbook, gives the recipe for Muesli, formulated by the Bircher-Benner Clinic and based on uncooked oatmeal. This formula was developed at the clinic as a result of trying to make a food as perfect as possible and containing all the ingredients of mother's milk. Elderly people tested on this formula have shown an increase in energy. Thousands of Swiss thrive on it. Mr. Hauser says: "Certainly it is a whole and natural food, superior to the tortured, denatured foods shot from guns and otherwise divorced from nature: milled, smashed, or rolled until nothing is left but pure starch."

The Muesli recipe: *1 tablespoon whole oats, 2 table-spoons water, juice of ½ lemon, 1 tablespoon rich cream, 2 apples and honey to taste. Soak the whole oats in the water overnight. In the morning add the lemon juice and cream and mix well. Wash but do not peel apples. Shred them into the oats and stir. Serve at once (10).*

Agnes Toms tells us in her excellent cookbook to cook oats in only enough water to cover, with salt added for taste, for 3 to 5 minutes. She says "Do not buy 'quick' oats, as additional mangling destroys much of the vita-min-B complex." She suggests adding sunflower seeds, polished rice powder or wheat germ to make a delectable hot cereal (11).

Lelord Kordel's cookbook gives a recipe for raw cracked-wheat cereal: *"Soak 2 cups of raw cracked wheat overnight in 4 cups of milk or fruit juice. Serves 4 athletes or 6 non-athletes."* (12)

Beatrice Trum Hunter reminds us that whole grains require longer cooking than cracked grains. In her cookbook she suggests slow baking with or without water, cooked in the deep well in a stove or a fuelless cooker overnight (an electric cooker or beanpot or a wide-mouth thermos can be used—see directions in her book). She also gives a mouthwatering recipe for a mixed cereal: *1 tablespoon sesame seeds, 1 tablespoon sunflower seeds, ½ cup whole wheat flour, ½ cup barley flour, ¼ cup rye flour, ¼ cup soy flour, ¼ cup cornmeal, ¼ cup brown rice, 1 teaspoon salt, 4 tablespoons honey, 4 tablespoons oil, 2 cups boiling water. Blend honey and*

*water and pour over mixture of dry ingredients. Mix
well; put into oiled casserole. Bake at 350 degrees about
30 minutes. Turn off heat but leave in oven to keep hot,
stirring occasionally, till all liquid has been absorbed*
(13).

Adelle Davis's cookbook (14) suggests uses for wheat
germ, the king of cereals. Since raw wheat germ is less
palatable, she suggests taking 4 cups of raw wheat germ,
adding ½ cup warmed honey, and spreading the mixture
in a shallow baking pan to bake at 300 degrees for 10
minutes. Cooled and refrigerated in a plastic bag it can
be broken up and used with milk as a cold cereal or
mixed with any other hot or cold cereal.

Fortunately, granola has caught on and many people
are eating it. It contains unprocessed nutritious goodies
and is delicious.

There are many other possibilities for using whole
grains as cereals. Millet, which looks a little like cornmeal, is the basic food of the Northern Chinese, who
count on it for energy. Scientists in the United States
have found that it is the only grain supplying many vitamins, with particularly high amounts of B-2 and
lecithin. It has been found to be non-acid-forming, non-
fattening, easily digested, and slightly laxative. This
cereal is the most ancient food of the human race, and
Pythagoras in 2500 B.C. advised his followers to use it to
improve health and strength. Millet is cooked like cornmeal, in water with a little salt to make a porridge or
used as a vegetable dish topped with butter. It is delicious. (Recipes for cooking millet may be found in the
cookbooks already mentioned.)

Whole brown rice (as opposed to the vitamin-robbed
white rice) is another choice for cereal, used with cream
or milk and honey, or served as the usual vegetable dish.
The macrobiotic brown rice is excellent. It is chewy and
nutty and simply delicious served with butter.

Cornmeal, like wheat, is now degerminated and the valuable corn germ, like the removed wheat germ—the most healthful part of the food—is missing in regular supermarket products. If you have some unused degerminated cornmeal you can add wheat germ to make up the deficit until you get whole natural cornmeal.

Other possibilities are wheat grits, brown rice grits, soy grits, rye grits, barley or buckwheat grits (also called groats) and bulgur. All of these, plus seven-grain cereal combinations—hot or cold—are available at health food stores which specialize in undegerminated, unprocessed, unrefined cereals. For those who do not have health food stores in their areas, there are excellent suppliers and millers who will mail you these products.

References

1. Fred D. Miller, D.D.S. *Open Door to Health*. New York, N.Y.: Arco Books, 1969.
2. Adelle Davis. *Let's Cook It Right*. New York, N.Y.: Harcourt Brace Jovanovich, 1962.
3. James Rorty and N. Phillip Norman, M.D. *Tomorrow's Food*. Old Greenwich, Conn.: Devin-Adair Co., 1956.
4. Ruth Bircher-Benner. *Eating Your Way to Health: The Bircher-Benner Approach to Nutrition*. Penguin Books, 1972.
5. *Open Door to Health*.
6. John Feltman "You Can Live without Sugar." *Organic Gardening and Farming*. October 1974.
7. Dr. Jean Mayer. From a statement made before the U.S. Senate Select Committee, Washington, D.C. 5 March 1973.
8. *National Enquirer*. 7 October 1974.
9. An Evening with Adelle Davis. Twelfth Annual International College of Applied Nutrition Symposium. 9 April 1972.

10. Gayelord Hauser. *The Gayelord Hauser Cookbook.* New York, N.Y.: G. P. Putnam's Sons, 1963.

11. Agnes Toms. *Eat, Drink and Be Healthy.* New York, N.Y.: Pyramid Publications, 1967.

12. Lelord Kordel. *Cook Right—Live Longer.* New York, N.Y.: Universal Publishing and Distributing, 1970.

13. Beatrice Trum Hunter. *The Natural Foods Cookbook.* New York, N.Y.: Pyramid Publications, 1967.

14. *Let's Cook It Right.*

Cell Salts and Beauty

A FRIEND called me recently to report that she had read of a formula, containing certain cell salts, designed to produce a good night's sleep. She had tried it and was surprised to find that it did, indeed, give her the promised good night's sleep. I looked up this formula in the book she had mentioned (1) and tried it myself. It worked for me, too. The formula was described as follows: "For the strange restlessness and the morbid, frightening dreams that follow radiation sickness, Calc. Phos., Calc. Fluor., Mag. Phos., and Kali. Mur., if taken in a little hot water and sipped upon retiring, will invariably act as a charm. The patient, falling into a restful sleep, will awaken to a new world in the morning."

These terms may sound like language used on Mars or some other distant planet. Actually, they are abbreviations for longer names which belong to the separate cell salts. What are cell salts? Can they be used for ordinary insomnia, not just that which follows radiation sickness? Can they be used for other disturbances also? Indeed, they are being used by a few enlightened people for all sorts of physical disturbances Although this is intended to tell you how they work for beauty, I will mention briefly their connection with health, because beauty depends upon good health. As you probably know by now my theme song is: *You cannot look well if you don't feel well.* After we discuss how the cell salts can improve beauty, if you wish to learn more about how they are improving health, I will tell you how to find this information.

What Are Cell Salts?

Cell salts are not drugs. They are tiny, sweet-tasting, white tablets about twice as thick as the head of a pin. They contain minerals that, on analysis, have been found already to exist in the body. They are considered necessary for proper growth and maintenance of health. For this reason they are known as biochemical cell salts, or the Schuessler cell salts, named after the physician who "discovered" them. There are twelve cell salts and they have the following names:

1. Calcarea Phosphorica (phosphate of lime), abbreviated as Calc. Phos.
2. Kali Phosphoricum (phosphate of potash or potassium) or Kali. Phos.
3. Magnesia Phosphorica (magnesium phosphate) or Mag. Phos.
4. Natrum Phosphoricum (phosphate of soda) or Nat. Phos.
5. Ferrum Phosphoricum (phosphate of iron) or Fer. Phos.
6. Natrum Sulphuricum (sulphate of soda) or Nat. Sulph.
7. Kali Sulphuricum (sulphate of potash) or Kali. Sulph.
8. Calcarea Sulphurica (sulphate of lime) or Calc. Sulph.
9. Kali Muriaticum (chloride of potash) or Kali. Mur.
10. Natrum Muriaticum (sodium chloride) or Nat. Mur.
11. Calcium Fluorica (fluoride of lime) or Calc. Fluor.
12. Silicea (silica)

These cell salts are not new, but merely ignored or forgotten in favor of drugs. They were "discovered" as early as 1873 by W. H. Schuessler, M.D. He analyzed human blood and isolated these important minerals, which are always found in human ashes after death, proving that they are an integral part of the body. In countless experiments, Dr. Schuessler learned that if any of the body cells become deficient in these minerals, the deficiency causes an abnormal or "diseased" condition. He ascertained by various symptoms which minerals were lacking in his patients, and supplied them. He found that if diseases are curable at all, and the proper cell salt is chosen and given in the proper amount, the deficiency that causes the abnormality is corrected, and the body heals itself. Thus the cell salts are not used to "cure" anything; they are merely supplied to the body to remedy a *deficiency* so that health can return to the cells, and thus to the body, which is made up of cells (2).

Mira Louise, the late Australian naturopath and nutritionist, who was a cell salt specialist, stated in her writings, "The action of these cell salts is little short of miraculous."

My Own Experience

Although I had mentioned the cell salts in my book, *Get Well Naturally* (3), and had taken a few of them now and then, I had never used them consistently. But after being reminded of them by my friend who used the insomnia formula, I decided to investigate them further. I read every word of the few books which describe their uses for various symptoms and became so intrigued I made a momentous decision—for me, at least. Although an advocate of vitamins and minerals for many years, I decided to give vitamins up for two whole weeks and substitute cell salt therapy just to see what would happen. Edgar Cayce had stated that one should give up vitamins for two weeks once or twice a year so that the body would not become too dependent on them. To date, I had never had the courage to try it, but now I decided to take the plunge.

Surprisingly, I did not fall apart on the cell salt program, though it is true that I made sure that my diet during that time was especially rich in food nutrients. Nevertheless, at the end of two weeks I was glad to get back to my vitamins, since they are necessary, also. Beyond a doubt, though, certain small symptoms which had refused to clear up were definitely helped by the cell salts. Since I am writing about beauty, I will report mainly the results relating to beauty.

Like most people these days, I had a few more falling hairs than I wanted. On the cell salt therapy, this falling of hair in my case began to slow down. My nails became longer and stronger and my skin, though already reasonably smooth, showed a bit more lustre. What really surprised me is that though I had reluctantly given up my natural iron supplement during the two weeks' experiment, my blood count, as judged by energy, nail and skin color, rose even higher on the cell salt Fer. Phos. (phosphate of iron).

The books listed at the end of this article state that certain cell salts influence specific skin problems. Since Calc. Sulph. is found in the skin, it contributes to skin health, according to the reports of J. B. Chapman, M.D. He also states that Kali. Sulph. aids in the formation of new skin, as well as aiding dry skin; that Calc. Phos. also aids dry skin, whereas Nat. Mur. helps excessively dry skin. He adds that Kali. Phos. is an aid for withered and wrinkled skin. Silicea is of paramount importance for skin (4).

For hair, there is help from the late Dr. Chapman as well as from his wife Esther, each of whom has written about the cell salts (5,6). Nat. Mur. is used for dry scalp and falling hair; Kali. Phos. is used as a help for falling hair too, as is Silicea, which is also suggested for brittle, ridged nails. And Calc. Phos. is mentioned in connection with hair which is already lost. For dandruff, Dr. Chapman lists Nat. Mur., Kali. Sulph. and Kali. Mur.

My own experience prompted me to ask a professional what he had observed about the effect of cell salts. He said, "Although I was dubious about their effect when I first began to work with cell salts, after witnessing near-miracles for nearly thirty years, I am now completely sold on them. Beauty-wise, my own wife suffered from splitting nails and falling hair. After she took the cell salt Silicea, her beauty operator asked her what had stopped her hair from falling and her nails from splitting. Her results took three months. She still takes Silicea as a preventive remedy."

Another professional told me that she had given the cell salts, in combination, to a group of college girls who were eating a very poor diet. On this therapy alone, their hair and nails definitely improved, taking about three months.

How Cell Salts Work

Why did the cell salts help my symptoms? Those of you who have read my book, *Secrets of Health and Beauty*, which includes my own health story, will remember that I was born with nutritional deficiencies (as many people are). I had corrected most of these through a rich nutritional diet—plus supplements. But the cell salts work differently from vitamins. Like all homeopathic remedies, they may be more effective in some cases because they are reduced to an almost infinitesimal degree of fineness, a process called "trituration." The first trituration is made by mixing one part of the mineral with nine parts of milk sugar, pounded in a mortar for two or three hours. This is called the "1x" potency. When one part of the 1x potency is mixed with nine parts of milk sugar and pulverized in the same way, it becomes the 2x potency and so on. Homeopathic potencies can reach the 200th potency, or higher, which reduces the particles to almost unbelievable fineness. But, by the same token, the cells of the body can accept and assimilate these fine particles, whereas they may reject or be unable to assimilate vitamins which are in grosser form. Since the cell salts are absorbed by the capillaries, they must be finer than capillaries. However, *both vitamins and cell salts are necessary*.

How to Take Cell Salts

Cell salts are not dependent on the usual method of digestion, so *they are not washed down with water*. They are assimilated by the body by osmosis, preferably via the saliva. Thus, they should be dissolved dry on or under the tongue, or dissolved in warm water and sipped slowly. The experts tell us that they should be taken in the 3x potency, except for Calc. Fluor., Nat. Mur., and Silicea, which should be in 6x potency.

Advised by experts, including the physicians who have written about cell salts, I took twenty-four tablets (six, four times daily) of the individual cell salts needed. If one were taking the entire combination in the tiny homeopathic tablets, the dosage of six tablets four times daily would still apply. If more than one individual remedy is taken, they can be alternated. Be sure to let them dissolve on your tongue. They may be taken between meals and at bedtime.

When I asked a professional expert if there is any danger in taking cell salts, he said, "Absolutely not! In agricultural chemistry we add the element most lacking in the soil, as a fertilizer to the soil. The plant picks up the element and recovers. The same law applies to the biochemic theory of the biochemic cell salts. If the reservoir of the human cell is already filled, there is no danger from taking the element, since the cell will merely reject it and it will be excreted from the body. Remember, cell salts are not drugs, but substances found in nature."

A combination of all the cell salts in balanced proprotions in one product has been developed by George W. Carey, M.D. This can be used as an adjunct to the individual cell salts, or as a preventive remedy.

Some people take the all-in-one salts, according to the label or, easier, a teaspoonful once a day. They then add the separate cell salts to supply their special needs, as described in the books listed below.

Some individuals have told me that they tried cell salts for two weeks without noticing any improvement. Cell salts are *not* drugs and usually do not work overnight! They slowly and subtly are rebuilt into your body to correct the mineral deficiencies and, according to Dr. Schuessler's research, the more deficient you are, the longer they may take. Then, like a good diet, they can become a way of life to prevent further mineral deficiencies.

Time for recovery resulting from the use of cell salts may vary from six weeks to three months, though Esther Chapman says, "But one does not need to wait for a full recovery to enjoy a measure of relief and greater ease." (7)

Cell salts are surprisingly inexpensive. Since they make wonderful companions to health foods and vitamins, health stores in Great Britain stock them as routinely as they do vitamins. In this country they are mainly available from homeopathic pharmacies and a few health stores. The books mentioned below can give you the information you need. (Please do not write me to ask which cell salt to use for which condition. As a reporter, I am not allowed to prescribe.)

Study the books on cell salts for yourself, particularly the one by J. B. Chapman, M.D.—a small, inexpensive treasure (8). You will find the information short, concise and intriguing, and I hope as rewarding for you as it has been for me.

References

1. Mira Louise. *More about Biochemistry.* (Out of print)
2. J. B. Chapman, M.D. *Dr. Schuessler's Biochemistry.* J. W. Cogswell, ed. St. Louis, Mo.: Formur International, 1975.
3. Linda Clark. *Get Well Naturally.* New York, N.Y.: Arco Books, 1968.
4. *Dr. Schuessler's Biochemistry.*
5. Ibid.
6. Esther Chapman. *How to Use the Twelve Tissue Salts.* New York, N.Y.: Pyramid Publications, 1971.
7. Ibid.
8. *Dr. Schuessler's Biochemistry.*

Body Regeneration

THE BODY is a marvelous factory. It also is a fantastic computer. Tests by radioactive tracers have shown that when certain natural organ substances are given to the body—let us say heart, liver, or kidney—those substances are delivered to the same areas in the body: heart to heart, liver to liver, kidney to kidney, to help regenerate the particular organ or gland which needs such help. More astonishing yet, if a *mixture* of organ substances is given the body, the body computer sorts out the separate ingredients and delivers them to the proper site.

There are various methods of rehabilitating the body cells, glands and organs. We have discussed how cell salts can rebuild cells by correcting deficiencies of certain minerals needed to keep them and the body in good working order. This method has worked for many who did not get the hoped-for results from the regular vitamin-mineral therapy. The reason is that the cell salts are so minute that the body can accept them more efficiently by osmosis, whereas vitamins and minerals may be rejected by a body, particularly if it is under par. An ailing body is not always able to assimilate the larger molecule of the necessary vitamin or mineral, whereas it may absorb the smaller molecule of the cell salts. An ideal arrangement is to use both.

Still another method of regenerating cells, glands and organs, is the Niehans method of injecting fresh cells, glands and organs from recently slaughtered animals into the human body. This method was originated by

Dr. Paul Niehans and is available in Europe at extremely high prices. Many miraculous recoveries have been credited to this type of therapy. There have also been some failures. One famous person told me that although it was reported that she had been helped by this treatment, she actually developed severe side effects. A man whom I know personally told me he received only a temporary improvement from the treatment. Later, when his health was again impaired, he tried a continuous program of good nutrition which included natural, fresh, organically raised food, plus a complete series of natural vitamin and mineral supplements. This, as a daily plan of living, keeps him in excellent condition, probably because it continues to supply his body with all it needs for continuous repair, rather than relying on a one-shot deal which may eventually be used up by the body.

Sometimes both approaches can be helpful: a massive treatment of certain substances to nudge sluggish glands and organs into activity once more, followed with a day-by-day supply of natural nutritional substances to feed, nourish and maintain the body. The explanation of why the Niehans treatment has been successful in many cases is that "impaired" glands apparently began to work again following stimulation through the fresh cell injection. It may also explain why massive amounts of synthetic vitamins, administered perhaps by injection by a physician, can accomplish similar results. There are nutritional physicians, however, who have discovered that if these massive amounts of certain synthetic vitamins are continued, they begin to act as drugs and over-stimulate the body, like whipping a tired horse. These physicians feel that even if a stimulating program is used at first, it should eventually be replaced by natural substances on a long-range basis. Only an expert is able to decide when the overstimulation point occurs. It differs from person to person.

Another method of stimulating inactive glands and organs toward normal is less drastic. It is the use of the protomorphogens, or cytotrophic extracts (as they are also known). Protomorphogens are protein substances extracted from the nucleic acids of a cell. When administered to patients, they proceed to the tissue of like substance and stimulate the cells of the organ or gland being treated to repair itself. Russian and American investigators have been studying the protomorphogens clinically and experimentally for over forty years. Bogolometz and co-workers have used the cytotrophic extracts for increasing the action of feeble, sick organs with definite success. Dr. Royal Lee and William A. Hanson have described investigative research work in a technical book, *Protomorphology: The Principles of Cell Auto Regulation.* This book is an academic masterpiece but much too difficult for the average layman to understand. So let me simplify here what the protomorphogens, or cytotrophic extracts, are and what they can apparently accomplish. The use of these extracts is not a do-it-yourself project; they are prescribed only in small amounts for gland or organ stimulation, by a doctor who understands them. Although they are used orally, too much can cause problems, whereas just the right amount has proved helpful in a variety of disturbances.

The cytotrophic extracts (protomorphogens) include extracts of veal bone, beef adrenals, brain, heart, kidney, lung, male and female sex organs, pancreas, parotid, pituitary, prostate, thymus, thyroid, uterus, eye and skin.

Alan H. Nittler, M.D., says, "I began using these substances in 1963. I am thoroughly convinced that they have power, some more than others. The heart extract has proved especially potent. One example involved a man about sixty years old. I was called to see him one evening because of severe precordial distress. I took him to my office, ran the heart function tests on him and discovered that he was having a heart attack. For a half hour I gave him, at intervals of five minutes, the heart cytotrophic extract plus vitamins C, E and B-2 plus niacinamide and B-6. The patient chewed these tablets and washed them down with water. Then the interval between dosages was lengthened to fifteen minutes for a couple of hours, then hourly for one week. He was awakened out of his sleep to take them. They were gradually decreased with the lessening of his pain, which finally disappeared entirely. After three months he returned to his occupation, which required him to climb a 150-step ladder to the exhaust system of a cement plant. He was able to do this several times daily without discomfort.

"I have many other similar case histories on file. However, my main use of the photomorphogens is not singly, but in combination in my detoxification and rebuilding program. I can truthfully say that my nutritional rehabilitation program for patients has definitely been more successful for the patients since I began the use of the cytotrophic extracts." (These substances are available *only* through doctors, who can order them for you from Standard Process Laboratories, 2023 West Wisconsin Avenue, Milwaukee, Wisconsin 53233. An M.D., D.O., D.C., N.D., or a dentist can get them for you.)

There is a related, simple and safe product that you can use at home, Malabar tablets and powder. This product contains cell units, extracted at low heat from internally defatted and defibered beef organ and glandular proteins. It includes a combination of pancreas, liver, brain, heart, duodenum and spleen substances. Derived from 100 percent pure organ meats, it can have no side effects. There is nothing else added, and it is a most carefully selected blend of inspected, healthy animal glandular tissues (organ meats). It is exsiccated, defatted and defibered and contains no fillers, milk, soya, casein, hydrolysates, coal tar, or sweeteners of any kind.

Because the fat is taken out of this product, the purines (uric acid-forming factors), the cholesterol, the DDT, stilbestrol (synthetic female hormone) and other undesirable factors or poisons are also eliminated, since they are stored in fatty tissues, including the liver. When the fat is removed, the hazard of the chemicals is also removed.

In this particular product, the fat is removed both internally and externally. With the fat and fiber extracted, the amount of protein is much higher. Also, with the fat and fiber removed, 99 percent of the digestive problem of any protein is eliminated, as often these two substances are the greatest cause of difficulty.

Because stilbestrol, along with pesticides and other poisons, settles in the fat of the liver and other organs, liver in its fresh form can be one of our worst foods today—even though it *should* be one of the best nutritionally. Since the protein product I have described is completely defatted, it does not present this problem, and therefore is an ideal way to use the organ meats under present-day circumstances.

Since there are no fillers in the product and nothing has been added, it has a protein content of 90 percent to 95 percent and contains the amino acids arginine, aspartic acid, glutamic acid, glycine, histidine, insoleucine, leucine, lysine, methionine, phenylalanine, threonine, valine and tryptophane. It also contains the natural B complex, being particularly high in vitamins B-12 and choline. *It takes more than 20 pounds of organ meats to make one pound of this protein mixture.* One physician has recommended taking ten tablets with each of three daily meals which contain other protein in some form. The powder can be mixed into a nutritious drink by combining two tablespoons of it with yogurt, lecithin and cherry concentrate for flavor—or with juices or milk. Recipes are available from the supplier on request.

When taking this product as well as any other concentrated protein, it is necessary to increase your calcium intake. The reason is that all animal protein products are high in phosphorus. The normal calcium-phosphorus ratio of food should be: $2\frac{1}{2}$ to 1. It is clear that if you raise the intake of phosphorus, the calcium should also be increased to maintain the normal ratio as nearly as possible. Otherwise symptoms of calcium deficiency can become apparent, the first of which may manifest as leg cramps. This principle applies to brewer's yeast, a high protein diet, or any other form of increased phosphorus in the diet. Merely add extra calcium as a precaution.

There are many success stories attributed to this protein food product. One woman described herself as "desperate." Although the doctor was doing all he could, nothing seemed to help her. She was besieged with allergies and a feeling of complete exhaustion, even though she was eating all the usual nutritionally recommended foods. She started using this glandular protein powder and reports that she began to notice improvement almost immediately. At first her husband objected to the cost of the product (because it is a quality product it is not sold at cut-rate prices), but when he saw the definite results in his wife, he began taking it himself and insisted that their two daughters follow suit. After two years on this therapy the wife has high vitality; her allergies have subsided; her skin and hair are also improved.

Others report that allergies are eventually dispelled by this glandular-organ food and, surprisingly, achievement of emotional balance is also mentioned by many who have used it. The greatest common benefit reported is increased energy. A high school athletic coach was overweight and lacked energy and vitality. He not only normalized his weight and blood pressure but gained the necessary energy and vitality for both his coaching activities and running a boys' summer camp. Impressed with the potential of the glandular-organ protein, he has made it a requirement of the diet of his athletes to build energy and endurance for the strenuous football and baseball seasons.

A woman who is a victim of hypoglycemia discovered that giving up starches and sugars and taking protein every three hours in some form made her feel better. When she substituted the glandular-organ protein powder, two heaping tablespoons three times daily in a drink, she noticed an improvement within a week's time, and she said, "I no longer had spells of anxiety."

A borderline diabetic also found it necessary to give up starches and sugars and rely upon proteins. She summed up her experience: "I found after consuming regular protein that it helped, but after two or three hours I would have a drop in energy and would become very irritable and weak mid-morning and mid-afternoon. I tried a protein drink at those times, but though it helped temporarily, not until I used the glandular-protein drink did I get a quick, sustained lift which carried me through to my next meal."

Thus, it is obvious, judging by the examples mentioned here, that if health is slipping, or if prevention of ill health is desired, there is hope in regenerating the body by means of a choice of the proper substances. This information is not new or a "fad," but has been proved over a long period of time. It is encouraging that such help is available.

Herb Magic

FOR YEARS people have used herbs for medicinal purposes. Every household in every country, in ages past, has had its favorite herbal remedies. Before this drug-laden era eclipsed herbs, doctors themselves used them. Today, however, in the more "civilized" countries, where herbs may well be a threat to commercial drug interests, herbs are being belittled just when the world's sickness rate is increasing and herbal therapy should be more useful than ever before. The Food and Drug Administration will not allow *any* statement of the curative value of *any* natural herb to appear on the label of a herb container. Thus, those of the younger generation who did not grow up learning the ancient heritage of herbal knowledge have no way of knowing which herb to use for a specific disturbance. What a pity!

Even animals know better. Bears, after winter hibernation, seek out certain herbs which they eat to strengthen their depleted forces. At the first hint of spring, honey bees use pollen for internal cleansing. Monkeys, living close to nature, have been known not only to eat certain herbs to cure themselves of certain illnesses, but also to carry these herbs to their companions who were too sick to hunt for themselves. Most amazing of all, crows and jackdaws, given poison by townspeople, have been able to find herbal antidotes to help them survive.

In Russia, more than a thousand herbs are used for curative purposes. The Chinese are encouraging the use of herbs for such diseases as gallstones, kidney inflammation, whooping cough, scarlet fever, mumps, cirrhosis of the liver, prolapsed uterus, typhoid, meningitis, encephalitis, influenza, pneumonia, tuberculosis, infectious hepatitis, some forms of dysentery, and hundreds of other ailments which have been known for centuries to yield to herbal treatment.

It is true that many drugs are derived from herbs. A search is under way for healing herbs on five continents by a veritable army of doctors and scientists. The difficulty is that when these herbs are brought back to the laboratory, they are not released to the public in natural form, but are synthesized. For example, natural aspirin (salicylic acid) was originally derived from willow bark and was presumably harmless. Today it is a chemical, a synthetic drug. Many un-hushed reports state that the synthetic aspirin can cause internal bleeding and other dangerous side effects. Penicillin is another example. Originally it was discovered in a mold on bread and oranges, also natural and presumably harmless. However, the demand for penicillin became so great that it, too, was synthesized. Although the antibiotic may have proved lifesaving to some, others have been so allergic to the synthetic version that they have died after a single injection in the doctor's office.

We are learning that it is folly to interfere with nature. Herbs, as both a natural medicine and a food, were evidently placed on earth to help sustain life.

The Bible says *(Genesis 1: 29, 30)*: "Behold, I give to you every herb bearing seed, which is on the surface of the entire earth, and every tree which has in it the fruit of a tree yielding seed. To you it shall be for meat. And to every beast of the earth and to every fowl of the air and to everything that creepeth upon the earth, wherein there is life, I have given every green herb for meat."

Why Do Herbs Help?

Those who claim that the value of herbs is an old wives' tale are merely uninformed. Many years ago, doubting Thomases cried "myth" when the American Indians insisted that a brew of pine needles would cure scurvy (now known as a disease due to vitamin-C deficiency). Later, a laboratory analysis found that pine needles were loaded with vitamin C, so the Indians were right, after all.

Euell Gibbons, a herb hunter and researcher, was puzzled as to why many herbs had been considered time-honored remedies. Finally he asked a university laboratory to analyze various species of herbs that he provided from his search in fields and forests. Sure enough, the laboratory found that the herbs contained substances which today we call vitamins and minerals. So the mystery of why herbs are helpful was solved, at least partially.

A New Herbal "Tonic"

Let me give you one example of the beneficial effects of herbs. Recently, I journeyed to Switzerland to investigate a herbal product I had been hearing much about. This product, used as a tonic, has had very little commercial publicity, yet the news of its good effects is spreading by word of mouth. I was anxious to learn why it is so popular.

The story begins with Frederick Pestalozzi, a Swiss engineer, who was confined to his bed with Méniere's disease. Unable to stand, walk, or hear, he was told by doctors that there was no hope. A friend suggested a herbal tonic as a last resort, and Fred Pestalozzi, believing there was nothing to lose after all else had failed, agreed to try it.

David Seymour, writing in the English *Evening Post*, said, "In three days he felt better. Three weeks later he walked again. Three months later he was back to work."

That was fifteen years ago. I can testify that Mr. Pestalozzi, now in his fifties, is well and strong and is still taking the herbal product. Furthermore, he is manufacturing it! After his health had returned, he approached Dr. Walter Strathmeyer, a German scientist, the originator of the tonic. Dr. Strathmeyer was interested not so much in making money as in helping people. Frederick Pestalozzi was also eager to make the tonic available to others. So Dr. Strathmeyer kept the German rights to his product (which is essentially the same, but carries a different name) and released the formula to Fred Pestalozzi to make and distribute to the rest of the world.

The Swiss factory, which I visited, is a credit to Fred Pestalozzi's engineering know-how. It is a neat, shining, compact building which houses modern stainless steel equipment designed to make and bottle the tonic without the touch of human hands. The number of bottles produced has mushroomed since the factory was built in 1961. In 1964, the laboratory produced 100,000 bottles as compared to 1967, when it produced 800,-000 bottles per five-day week, and shipped to 35 countries.

The English newspaper, *News of the World* (7 July 1968), reported that the benefits of this herbal tonic have been discovered by such people as Jack McClelland, channel swimmer, Sir Stanley Matthews, Mrs. Indira Ghandi, Gloria Swanson and Barbara Cartland, London's novelist and nutrition and beauty expert.

Briefly, the formula is a special type of yeast to which has been added carefully selected herbs, chosen to benefit every part of the body.

Documented Effects on Animals

The efficiency of this herb-fed yeast, as well as the absence of any harmful effects, has been proved in seven-year tests at the University of Zurich, Switzerland. The elixir has been fed to animals, with excellent results:

In one study lasting three-and-one-half years, rats fed this herbal mixture during their whole life span showed excellent results, with no side effects, when tested for growth, blood, cardiac activity and physical performance.

Another scientific study with mice revealed that some protection against radiation was evident.

The elixir was used in a veterinary test with seventy hens which had stopped laying. On the third day after the hens were given the herbal mixture, the egg yield rose daily from two, three and four eggs at the start, to fifteen per day at the end of the first week. In the third week the yield had climbed to twenty-four to twenty-six eggs a day, or a 50 percent increase.

A Doberman pinscher dog was unable to walk, due to lameness of her hindquarters. After four months on the herbal tonic she was again able to walk. A greyhound which had been regularly fed the herbal tonic won ten first places and eighteen second places in races in the last two years. Various race horses in Switzerland, when fed the tonic, also showed excellent performance records.

A picture shows a dachshund, four-and-a-half years old, also afflicted with paralysis of the hindquarters, a condition which had lasted two months. A second picture taken three weeks later, after the same herbal therapy, shows the dog running and playing like a puppy. A year later the dog was still free of paralysis.

In my opinion, the most dramatic response in animals was that of a boxer, ten years old. The "before" picture shows the dog with eczema, loss of hair, lassitude and dull eyes. The condition had existed for nine months and all other therapy had failed. After only six weeks on the herbal elixir, the dog is shown with bright and shining eyes, eczema gone, a growth of new, lustrous hair, and apparent revitalization.

Documented Effects on People

The herbal yeast supplement has accomplished these results in people:

Dr. Else Mann is a European general practitioner in an area which is usually cavity prone. She had previously tried a wide variety of calcium preparations, vitamins, even topically applied fluoride to combat the problem in her patients, with no appreciable results. After administering the herbal supplement in the form of drops to pregnant women as well as to children of various ages, she noted an 87.5 percent drop in caries, which later became 100 percent. She also witnessed additional benefits: resistance to rickets, children's complaints and catarrhal disorders. Delicate and sickness-prone children became stronger and put on weight. No undesirable side effects were apparent.

At the University of Hamburg, a clinical investigation of 2000 children revealed that more than half of the children suffered from nervous disorders. A high percentage suffered from lack of appetite, insomnia, inability to concentrate, weak memory and lack of initiative. All disturbances were improved by administration of the herbal tonic, and personality problems improved as well. These experiments were repeated several times in close cooperation with doctors.

Dr. Rohling, (M.D.), chief medical officer of a European biological sanatorium, prescribed this same herbal tonic for 3000 patients. He reports improvement in blood circulation disturbances, including high and low blood pressure, vascular spasm and rheumatic disorders, and complete remission of eczema and psoriasis—in some cases with no relapse after as long as eight years. He also noted relief from insomnia and anemia.

Dr. Rohling states, "In the whole of my medical practice, covering a period of twenty-two years, I have encountered no preparation having the same range and degree of efficacy as this herbal supplement."

In a Swiss institute for mentally defective children, Karl Suter, M.D., reported improvement in the mental development, as well as the emotional and temperamental condition, of the children. Longstanding cases of bedwetting, hostility and aggression were also markedly improved.

Dr. Suter says, "In contrast to so many other medical preparations, this supplement is absolutely harmless and can be administered with confidence in any circumstances."

Other physicians have noticed resistance to infectious diseases, better sleep and relief from constipation after use of the supplement.

I have "before" and "after" pictures of a child whose face was covered with eczema before being treated orally with the herbal drops. Two months later the skin condition was almost entirely reversed and smooth once more.

I also have a signed testimonial from a woman suffering from diabetes. She wrote, "I have been taking a great variety of tonics which I had to abandon because my blood sugar increased considerably. My doctor prescribed the herbal drops. Although I take them regularly, my blood sugar remains unchanged and normal."

A final report I have chosen is that of the effect of the herbal tonic on chronic corneal herpes, an eye complaint recognized to be one of the most difficult to cure in the entire field of ophthalmology. David Pestalozzi, M.D., head of the Eye Department of Cantonal Hospital in Olten, Switzerland, tried the herbal tonic in three cases of this serious affliction. He writes, "In all three cases, after administration of the herbal yeast elixir in addition to the therapy previously practiced, the condition cleared and there was no further relapse."

Cosmetic effects of this herbal mixture have also been noticed. One woman, whose statements were verified by her hair dresser and manicurist, reported that her hair gained new life and "bounce" and her nails, which had been not only brittle and delicate, but yellow like those of a heavy smoker, became long and hard, and the new nail growth was normal in color. Colored pictures also testify to this.

Others report that new hair growth is often noted, though sometimes there is a temporary loss of the old hair to make way for the new.

The original herbal yeast tonic, called an elixir because it was in liquid form, combined yeast on which was grown ninety-four herbs (chosen because each herb has long been known to help some part of the body) plus honey, malt and orange juice. Unfortunately, there was difficulty in importing this elixir (although there are recent assurances that its import will be facilitated). European doctors also found that at least four bottles were needed to bring optimum results. However, there is recent good news.

The same product, made by the same manufacturer, is now available in tablet form, which is easier and more convenient for many. There is actual improvement for some people over the effects of the elixir. There is no sweetening added, so diabetics or hypoglycemics can take it. Another exciting feature of the tablets is that instead of the original type of yeast used (torula or *Candida utilis*) an improved and unusual type of yeast has been substituted with excellent results. This yeast is the well known primary yeast, known as *Saccaromyces cerovisiae*, but with a difference. This particular yeast has not been heat-killed, as is the usual nutritional yeast, nor is it alive, as in baking yeast which has been found to gobble up your own supply of B vitamins. Instead, this yeast is in an in-between state, or *active*! This means that because it has been dried at body temperature for only fifteen hours, it still contains all of the enzymes, which help both its assimilation and digestion.

There are no additives, chemicals, or preservatives present. The number of herbs has been reduced from ninety-four, as in the elixir, to seventeen. These are in homeopathic form and have been carefully selected to include those which are compatible, not only to each other, but to the body. Again, however, as in the elixir, they have been chosen to aid various functions in the body. I have a list of these herbal functions before me, but due to the restrictions in labeling in the United States, neither the manufacturer nor I are allowed to give out this information. But no matter, the herbs are there, their names are listed on the label of the tablet container, and they are included to help you whether you know what they do, or not. In addition to the benefits of the herbs, the yeast itself provides RNA, B vitamins, amino acids (protein factors) as well as the enzymes mentioned earlier. This is important, because yeast and body cells both need oxygen to reproduce cells, and the tablets contain everything necessary to contribute health to the body cells.

Both the elixir and the tablets are called Bio-Strath. The Bio-Strath products are already the rage in Europe and Scandinavian countries, and since the Bio-Strath tablets have become available in this country, there are hundreds of enthusiastic unsolicited testimonials about them, including mine. In general, laboratory test reports from European countries, including Switzerland and England, reveal that with animals, the Bio-Strath products significantly increase the natural resistance of the body.

In the tablets, the added protective factor derived from the cerovisiae yeast may enhance this factor.

In reading over some of the unsolicited testimonials from people in this country who have been using the Bio-Strath tablets, I find repeated mention of improvement with digestion, colds, strep infections, increase of vitality, and even stimulation of hair growth. One of my friends, whose hair was previously patchy and thin, after using the tablets showed me her hair which is now thick, healthy, and grows so vigorously she has to have it cut every two weeks.

Most people take the tablets at the rate of one before each meal.

Ginseng: Fact or Fancy?

GINSENG has been the "in thing" now for some time especially in California and particularly in Hollywood where health stores are selling it as fast as they can get it.

In an article titled "Hollywood Stars Flip for Red Chinese Aphrodisiac," Alfred E. Stone wrote that bottles containing 150 eight-gram capsules of ginseng cost between $15 and $25. The average price, he says, was $20 but he predicts an even higher cost.

The natural question is: Is all this excitement warranted or merely a figment of someone's imagination?

I have done research on ginseng for a full year, collecting every shred of documented information I could find. I will share this information with you and let you decide for yourself.

I will tell you one thing: the Food and Drug Administration has been quite unhappy about the whole thing, jumping on ginseng distributors and health stores alike for making claims about it. I am neither making claims, endorsing or criticizing it. I am merely reporting the facts as I found them.

What Is Ginseng?

Ginseng grows in secluded areas, thrives only in special soil, brings up all the minerals from that soil and should be harvested only after six years or longer. In fact, there is belief that the older the roots, the more potent. Richard Lucas writes, "For over 5,000 years, 400 million Chinese and Koreans, each of many generations, have steadfastly maintained that ginseng had great merit as a remedy in a variety of ills. It would be foolish to suppose that for fifty centuries the Chinese were basing their faith in ginseng on nothing but sheer superstition."(1)

The Chinese who can afford it use ginseng for cure of disease as well as for prevention of illness. They particularly stress the fact that ginseng is a factor in virility, which may account for the fact that they have been able to procreate children at the ages of sixty, seventy and over, a possible effect of ginseng upon the endocrine glands. At any rate ginseng is considered so valuable by the Chinese that at one time Imperial ginseng sold for $3,200 per pound.

Lucas states that ginseng apparently acts as a rejuvenator and reactivates the sexual organs as well as the endocrine glands, which in turn control the body function, and the assimilation of vitamins and minerals.

What Other Countries Say about It

He reports that the Institute of Experimental Medicine in Russia is devoting much research to ginseng. At first They kept their findings secret and appropriated the entire supply of Korean ginseng, valued at $120 million dollars. Later they planted their own supply in huge plantations in South Siberia. They finally announced a few of their discoveries in connection with the use of ginseng: "It strengthens the heart, the nervous system, and increases the body's manufacture of hormones."

According to Joseph E. Meyer, ginseng was an official drug in the United States Pharmacopoeia from 1840 to 1880 (2). At present it is listed among the unofficial drug-plants (on page 51) of Bulletin No. 89, U.S. Department of Agriculture, Bureau of Plant Industry.

Wild ginseng sells for a higher price than the cultivated. Lucas explains why: "It is believed that the rejuvenating action of ginseng on the sex glands is due to certain radioactive substances that it absorbs from the soil. Being of organic origin, these radioactive substances are beneficial rather than harmful and are *unlike* the strontium 90 and other *inorganic* fallout products. It is assumed that the wild plant is more potent because it selects its own location and chooses the soil where the organic (natural) radioactivity is the highest."

Wild ginseng was previously used in early America by Indian medicine men.

What's Good about Ginseng?

The Chinese, Japanese and Koreans believe that ginseng is a panacea. But what about non-Oriental researchers? Are they as enthusiastic?

A. R. Harding, M.D., wrote that in various ailments from which his patients suffered, they recovered more quickly with ginseng than with any other form of medicine or treatment (3). He became so impressed with ginseng that he gave up his medical practice and spent the rest of his life studying ginseng and presenting his findings in his book.

Dr. Harding gives some examples. He tried ginseng on a middle-aged man with rheumatism, for which the man had tried everything else without success. When Dr. Harding added ginseng to his treatment, the man recovered.

Dr. Harding also found that ginseng stimulated a healthy flow of digestive juices and said that ginseng combined with the juice of a ripe pineapple is a treatment for indigestion *par excellence*. He writes: "This combination stimulates the healthy secretion of pepsin, thereby insuring good digestion without requiring the usual pills to relieve fullness and distress so common to the American people."

Dr. Harding prescribed ginseng tea for the chronic

cough of another patient who took it with meals and between meals. In two weeks, the cough was gone. He adds: "It would take too long to enumerate the ailments I have cured with ginseng; but I think it will suffice to say that I have cured every case where I have used it with one exception: a case of consumption in the last stages. Even so the lady and her husband both told me it was the only medicine she took during her illness that did her any good ... If a disease can be cured, ginseng will cure it where no drug will."

A California doctor, an M.D., whose name I am purposely deleting in order to protect him from a deluge of mail, found a more complete analysis of ginseng in the German professional journal, *Apothekerpost*, 1954. This analysis revealed that ginseng includes saponines, etheric oils, panacen and panax acid (fatty acids, the names meaning "panacea"), vitamins B-1 and B-2 as well as the minerals phosphorus, iron, aluminum, copper, manganese, cobalt, and the main element, sulfur. There are also a few enzymes present such as amylase and proteolytic enzymes.

This physician conducted his own research and later gave ginseng to his patients. He got it from the Chinatown district of the large city in which he practices. He learned that ginseng can help the following conditions in some cases:

- Heart—oppressed breathing, chest tightness, fast heart beat, sudden palpitations, especially when sitting
- Creaking in joints, neck and vertebral joints of the cervical spine. Weak knees and tottering, cramp-like pain from right knee joint down to toes; rheumatism, gout; sciatic neuritis
- Skin—itching and pimples on neck and chest
- Stomach pain, diarrhea and uric acid

- Nervous prostration and general weakness. Nervous exhaustion
- Tiredness in limbs, tremor, poor circulation, cold hands and feet
- Eyes—double vision, spots before eyes
- Heartburn with thirst
- Stinging pain in liver and bilious diarrhea
- Frequency of urination
- Sexual weakness, impotency and irritation

This physician adds that ginseng can also be used for hepatitis, atherosclerosis, forgetfulness and all conditions where constitutional weakness or degeneration in the aging process is noted. He finds it also helpful for throat symptoms, dry pharyngitis and the speaking and singing voice. For his patients, he makes a tincture from raw materials found in his local Chinatown. He tells of three case histories resulting from the use of ginseng:

1. An eighty-year-old man was suffering from depression, restlessness and brain fog. He recovered immediately from these symptoms but saw no results as an aphrodisiac.
2. A middle-aged woman was menopausal, depressed, lacked energy and exhibited sexual indifference. She took one teaspoon of elixir of ginseng twice daily. Her energy increased, her depression disappeared and she reported that she sparkled again. Her sexual indifference remained unchanged.
3. A fifty-year-old man experienced a return of energy and a marked diuresis (release of stored water from the body).

The physician believes that ginseng is the closest that we can come to a panacea, and that it is not accidental that it has been successful for 2,000 years in improving health. However, his most surprising findings are that ginseng helps reverse graying and loss of hair (he says that ginseng added to alcohol is a helpful hair lotion); and most exciting, he has found ginseng is an antidote for narcotic and drug addiction! He feels that this may prove to be one of its greatest contributions.

There are assorted other disturbances which apparently respond to ginseng. The Australians, who use North Korean ginseng, believe that the herb helps to regulate blood pressure and prevent arteriosclerosis; improves digestion and assimilation; relieves constipation and inflammation of the urinary tract; aids lung trouble; helps recovery from fatigue and enervating illness; and perpetuates youthfulness and virility.

Dr. Finn Sandberg, professor of pharmacognosy at the University of Upsala, Sweden, tested ginseng in a double-blind experiment with students. The test lasted thirty-three days and the results, according to Dr. Sandberg, showed a statistically significant increase in mental concentration, psychomotor activity and simultaneous capacity. Dr. Karl-Heinz Ruekert, of Switzerland, has presented data showing that ginseng greatly improved the swimming performance of mice. This experiment lasted for twenty-one days (4).

An Oriental business executive, who has watched the effect of ginseng in his own country, states that ginseng works slowly to rebuild the body. He finds that it has been helpful for insomnia, some types of ulcers and apparently eliminates alcohol from the system. It may give relief for arthritis, he says, but is a definite help for diabetic patients, who of course should check with their physicians about using it. He, too, has seen improvement in hair growth and reversal of graying hair. He also says bones heal faster, hearing improves and Orientals avoid aches and pains of old age.

Maxine Block interviewed many stars about their experiences with ginseng. George Maharis, Clint Walker,

Cary Grant, Mae West, Glenn Ford, Shelley Winters, John Wayne, Burl Ives and others admitted taking ginseng because of its tonic effect.

According to Miss Block, Gisele Mackenzie says: "My father was a doctor. He stressed natural vitamins. I think of ginseng as a vitamin and drink it (as a tea) as hot as can be borne before lunch and dinner. This pleasant aromatic tea stimulates the nervous system. Since it is a natural herb and not a synthetic drug, it cannot harm the body" (5).

How to Take Ginseng

There are various ways to take ginseng. Some take it in powder form, contained in capsules. Others drink it as a tea or chew the root itself. Still others, as the doctor I mentioned previously, use it in the form of an elixir, measured by drops or teaspoonfuls. (The formula for making the elixir, incidentally, appears in Richard Lucas' book, *Nature's Medicines* (6).) A source for the elixir in the United States is now available (7).

Orientals suggest one very important precaution: do not take pineapple, tomato, grapefruit, lemon, orange, carrot or turnip or vitamin C until three hours *after* taking the ginseng. These fruits, foods or vitamin C neutralize the effect of the food value of the herbs, they believe.

Do these herbs, ginseng in particular, always do the job? Peter Lupus, TV star of *Mission Impossible*, is quoted by Maxine Block as saying: "I have no qualms about testifying for ginseng. I consider it a rejuvenator, an invigorator, a reactivator. It's also supposed to be a good aphrodisiac. But one thing you must remember: you can't just brew a cup or take a single capsule and say, 'Man, now I feel great.' A studio pal tried it for two days and reported that he didn't see any difference in how he felt. You have to keep on taking ginseng. You can't expect to use it for a week and see a miracle."

Some people take ginseng once a day to stay healthy; others take it twice—once in the morning and once at night. Some people feel a lift fifteen minutes after taking a cup of tea but I am not one of them; I get an almost immediate pickup from taking a capsule of American ginseng, dissolved in a cup of boiling water. So we all differ.

Most people claim there are no side effects, either. But, some people cannot take American ginseng at night because it is too stimulating. Tea from a tea tab, on the other hand, which can be taken at night, seems to overcome insomnia for many.

There is some controversy about ginseng. A health store owner, on hearing of the great benefits of taking ginseng, ordered it in the form of tea bags. He and an assistant took it religiously, but showed no results. It turned out to be a "cull" of some ginseng from which most of the strength had been removed before shipping it to this country. For this reason I urge both health store owners and customers to evaluate objectively the ginseng they buy.

Although I and willing helpers tested various types of ginseng, obviously we could not test them all. However, (and this is important) the individual difference of each person should be considered. Some types of ginseng are too stimulating for some people; other types may not be stimulating enough or need to be taken in greater amounts for a longer time to get results. Since there are many good sources of ginseng, the proof of the pudding is in the taking.

Ginseng is not actually a drug. It is a vitamin-mineral-rich food. It may or may not be for you. The only way you can find out is to give it a fair trial—providing your pocketbook can stand it!

References

1. Richard Lucas. *Nature's Medicines*. New York, N.Y.: Universal Publishing and Distributing Corp., 1968.

2. Joseph E. Meyer. *The Herbalist*. New York, N.Y.: Sterling Publishing Co., Inc., rev. ed. 1968.

3. A. R. Harding, M.D. *Ginseng and Other Medicinal Plants*. Columbus, Ohio: Fur-Fish-Game, rev. ed. 1972.

4. *Here's Health* (English magazine). January 1975.

5. Maxine Block. "How the Stars Stay Forever Young and Beautiful." *Hollywood Magazine*. May 1970.

6. *Nature's Medicines*.

7. An elixir in a liquid yeast base is available from The Three Sheaves, 16 Hudson Street, New York, N.Y. 10013.

Is Yogurt Safe?

A READER has written: "Would you please clear up a worrisome thing for me and others? I have used yogurt, on and off, for years, and my health has seemed better for it. However, a friend brought me some published material which said that yogurt causes cataracts as well as a vitamin B-2 deficiency. I don't have cataracts, but is this information true? Something which has been used for hundreds of years can't be all bad. Can you clarify this for me and others?"

The published material you probably referred to appeared mid-1970(1), when a news release from Johns Hopkins School of Medicine stated that rats fed *exclusively* on a commercial yogurt diet developed cataracts, due to galactose (one ingredient in milk sugar). Soon afterward, an article appeared in *Let's Live* magazine, presenting some European research, plus some unsubstantiated personal opinions of the author, and the controversy was on. The article challenged the Johns Hopkins findings and stated that yogurt could be good or bad, depending on the source, the type and the way it was made, and then added some further opinions for which so far there is no documentation or proof.

As a reporter I try to document the sources of any information I report. So I will try to clear up the confusion about yogurt, not with my own opinions (although I do eat yogurt), but with the findings of scientific investigators, who may be right or wrong, but are sincere in their efforts.

Yogurt is made, as you know, from milk to which a

culture has been added. The culture grows and multiplies like yeast cells in bread making, until the milk becomes slightly tart and custard-like. Those manufacturers who use a uniform method and a superior culture usually get a uniform product, whereas those who make their own yogurt may get variable results from batch to batch. Even the flavor in separate containers in the same batch of homemade yogurt may vary. Before yogurt became so common in the United States, a friend of the late Eleanor Roosevelt told me that Mrs. Roosevelt had it made for her by a private supplier. Before she boarded a ship for Europe she sampled various small containers of a batch of the yogurt, especially made for her, and chose the one with the flavor she preferred. From this container an entire new batch was made so that Mrs. Roosevelt could take it with her to eat on shipboard.

Today, now that yogurt is so common, there are many varieties to choose from. This does not mean that *any* yogurt is a magical food just because it bears the name. Like any other food, it should be chosen with discrimination. If yogurt is made from questionable milk sources, old or pre-soured, or is embellished with synthetic flavors, sugary fruits, and artificial colorings, the product is not going to be the equivalent of the yogurt which originated in various European countries, and is believed by many investigators (among them, Professor Elie Metchnikoff, of the Pasteur Institute in France) to be responsible for their health and longevity. After all, yogurt is a delicate food, and should be chosen, or made, with tender loving care.

Why Take Yogurt?

There are many kinds of bacteria in the world, good and bad. Many people assume that if it is called "bacteria" it is dangerous, but this is not true; the term is used for both types. Our intestines, for example, can have disturbing bacteria which can result in digestive disturbances: gas, cramps, putrefaction, auto-intoxication, etc. Salmonella is an example of a disturbing bacteria. But there can be, and should be, *friendly* bacteria in the colon which can help vanquish the unfriendly types of bacteria and help promote health. If the right substances are fed the body, the friendly bacteria, known as the "intestinal flora," can increase and provide protection against the undesirable bacteria. Yogurt contains the culture which can populate the intestines with billions of these friendly microorganisms or bacteria. When the flora is kept in optimum condition, it can encourage better digestion and better elimination. Some doctors prescribe it for constipation. But it can do much more.

Biologists tell us that the intestines should also have some acid, and yogurt (or other forms of soured milks) can help provide this valuable lactic acid needed by the stomach for digestion, which is protection against infection (unwanted germs cannot live in an acid medium) (2). Acid is also needed for assimilation of calcium, iron, and protein. Many scientists believe that lactic acid is the only acid which has healing properties. Yogurt can also help the intestinal flora to manufacture free vitamins for you: the B complex, especially niacin, riboflavin (B-2), biotin and folic acid as well as vitamin K (3).

One of the greatest benefits of yogurt, however, is little known. It is a *natural* antibiotic. An eight-ounce jar of seven-day-old yogurt has been found to contain the equivalent of fourteen penicillin units (4). And in a Turkish study, yogurt was found to destroy two types of human TB and one type of bovine TB. This has been proved on animals which were completely free of infection from five to twelve hours after being fed yogurt (5). Certain pathogenic microorganisms have also been fed yogurt itself. The whey in yogurt kills amoeba in five minutes. In World War I, yogurt cured amoebic dysentery in humans when used in enemas. In one hour the typhus organism is killed as well as S. paratyphus, Br. abortus, V. Comma, E. Subtilis; in two hours the S. pullorum, S. dysentariae, P. vulgaris, M. pyrogenes; in five hours E. coli, K. pneumonia, also streptococcus and staphylococcus; and in 24 hours, L. lactis, C. diphtheriae, S. mitis, S. fecalis. Many bacteriological experiments have shown the power of yogurt bacteria to hinder the development of these and other pathogenic organisms. Thus science has proved yogurt to be an invaluable natural antibiotic (6).

Antibiotic drugs kill good as well as bad bacteria in the intestinal flora, throwing the body into a defenseless condition. For this reason, in Italy, doctors automatically prescribe yogurt simultaneously with antibiotic drugs to prevent the destruction of the valuable flora. Some people who are deficient in B vitamins develop no unfavorable symptoms until they are given antibiotic drugs (7). Yogurt can remedy such a state.

Yogurt culture was originally brought to America from Europe by the famous Rosell Institute of the La Trappe Monastery in Canada, knowing that some European countries have thrived for centuries on certain soured milks, of which yogurt and a sister product, kefir, are the most popular. Statistics show that approximately 80 percent of the diet of the people of the Caucasus region and the Balkan states is made up of cultured milk. A 1970 census placed the number of the people of the Caucasus who are *over 100 years of age* at 4,500 to 5,000. Of these 1,844 live in Georgia, or 39 per 100,000 of population; 2,500 live in Azerbaijan, or 63 per 100,000. In the United States, by comparison, the figure is only about three centenarians per 100,000 population (8).

We are fortunate in the United States to have a family from the Balkans who have been specialists in the preparation of yogurt and kefir and acidophilus culture for seven generations. Vasa Cubalevic, and his family, are responsible for the yogurt and kefir for the Alta Dena Dairy in California. Vasa Cubalevic is now making in this country the same strains of yogurt for which he was given an award of merit by King Peter II, of Yugoslavia, in 1940. I have a copy of this award before me. Vasa, as he is called, came to the United States in 1955 and has been head of the Continental Culture Specialties, in Glendale, California, ever since.

The culture used in yogurt varies with the manufacturer. The most common bacilli used in various soured milks are lactobacillus Bulgaricus, lactobacillus Caucasicus, lactobacillus bifidus. S. Termophilus and Bulgaricus are the most common strains used in this country. However, the lactobacillus Bulgaricus is extremely fragile and is sensitive to changes in the culture medium and can quickly lose its power to coagulate milk. This means that such a commercial starter cannot be perpetuated in homemade yogurt forever by using some of the previous batch to start a new one. The culture medium may not only lose its power but the food bacteria will become so low that the culture will become absolutely worthless. Even old laboratory cultures must be regenerated in a proper medium in order to produce an acceptable product. Yogurt (and kefir) found in health stores are usually the most reliable sources of properly cultured milk. If they are flavored with fruits or other flavorings, these additions should be natural, not synthetic, since the culture may continue to "feed" on such synthetic additives, including artificial coloring and sugar, which might pervert the product. This is why, as I have said before, that just because the product is stamped with the name "yogurt" does not guarantee that it is the same as that on which Europeans have lived, and thrived, for centuries.

119

Those manufacturers who are known for their integrity can be depended upon to provide you with a dependable yogurt. The Continental Culture specialists, for example, take pride in duplicating the methods used in the Balkans for generations. It is to them that I turned to find the answers to the bothersome question, will yogurt cause cataracts? Vasa Cubalevic may well be the most knowledgeable man on the subject of cultured milks in the United States. He provided the following answer to the cataract question.

A surprisingly large portion of the world cannot digest lactose (milk sugar). This group includes Africans, Colombian Indians (as well as our own Navajo Indians), Orientals and Eskimos. The reason for this is that these nationalities, after weaning, do not drink milk, largely because it is not available, and their bodies lose the function of the enzyme *lactase*, which is needed to digest *lactose* (milk sugar). When this happens, physical disturbances can follow the use of milk. For example, Navajo Indians reject American powdered milk because it gives them diarrhea. Milk is about 40 percent lactose, whereas yogurt contains only a trace. However, the Johns Hopkins rats were given a straight diet of commercial yogurt (they ate nothing else) and *rats also do not have the ability to digest lactose.*

The yogurt fed the rats contained a high ratio of galactose, a simple molecule in milk sugar, which the researchers blamed for the resulting cataracts. Actually, apparently no one thought about the inability of the rats to digest these substances. Furthermore, though the findings of the study were reported in 1970, it turned out later that these studies were not recent but had been conducted fifteen years earlier(9).

Vasa Cubalevic states that in the Caucasus and Balkan areas where yogurt and kefir have been consumed daily in great amounts, *there has never been any report of cataracts.*

Now what about that B-2 (riboflavin) deficiency supposedly caused by yogurt? Other findings state that cataracts can develop because of a deficiency of vitamin B-2 or the amino acid, tryptophane. There appears to be some substance to this theory, though before I give it to you, it is well to note that many ophthalmologists claim that there are different kinds of cataracts, produced by different causes: radioactivity, tension, calcium or protein abnormalities. So it is not safe to generalize that there is one single cause of cataracts, including yogurt, since this is not so.

It is true that there is a scientific report that galactose (a milk sugar molecule) is an antagonist of and can cause a deficiency of vitamin B-2(10). According to Dr. P. S. Day, of Columbia University, he found that a lack of vitamin B-2 can cause cataracts in both animals and humans. In fact, Dr. Sydenstricker, of the University of Georgia Hospital, treated many cases of opacities with 15 mgs of B-2 daily, and though it took nine months, the opacities were reversed. If the B-2 deficient diet was repeated, the opacities returned(11). However, this apparently applies to some people only. I have witnessed two people with cataracts who used the 15 mgs of B-2 faithfully for nine months and did not have success, as confirmed by an ophthalmologist. More cases are necessary for proof, and generalization is also dangerous. So it is possible that a high content of galactose might indeed create a deficiency of vitamin B-2 which might lead to cataracts *in some people*(12). Where does this high ratio of galactose come from?

Vasa Cubalevic believes that yogurt made as it was in the old countries should be made from whole, not fat-free, milk. But in this country people are so afraid of fat that whole milk has become an unproved no-no. So, since fat-free milk causes a watery yogurt, some manufacturers thicken it with powdered milk. This increases the ratio of galactose to a higher percentage. Now hear this: In the Johns Hopkins study, the rats were first given a combination of yogurt *and* a stock diet and developed no cataracts! But when they were switched to an exclusive diet of yogurt, which was found to contain 24 percent galactose, the cataracts appeared. The dry milk, added to yogurt, also increases its alkalinity which in turn contributes to a B-2 deficiency (13). So it may be preferable to use naturally richer milk to make your own yogurt than to add large amounts of powdered milk to watery non-fat milk. Continental Culture gets their delightful thick, creamy consistency with either whole or low-fat milk, *not* no-fat milk. If any manufacturer who has the proper testing equipment does add powdered milk, the amount can be kept below the questionable danger point. If the ratio of galactose is low, the yogurt will feed on it and reduce it by converting it to lactic acid.

If you are concerned whether or not you have a riboflavin deficiency, there are well known symptoms which appear long before cataracts: itchy reddened eye corners and a feeling of sand beneath the eye lids. Taking a generous amount of foods containing the B complex, which includes B-2 (liver and brewer's yeast are excellent sources), should help correct the deficiency. And, strangely enough, if you get enough of the right type of cultured yogurt, it will help you manufacture your own B-2 in your intestinal tract! Also, people with a milk intolerance appear to tolerate yogurt better, due to its acid. There is further information about causes and natural treatments of cataracts in one of my books (14).

The lactobacillus Bulgaricus helps to break down or predigest albumin, a protein found in milk and egg white. Once in the stomach the lactic acid assists the body in assimilating the protein. Furthermore, it converts lactose to lactic acid which helps people with an intolerance to lactose. What is more important is that once the Bulgaricus, Acidophilus and Caucasicus bacteria establish themselves as part of the intestinal flora, they continue to maintain their existence by feeding on any additional lactose that may be present in the body unless killed by antibiotics. People of Syria consume large quantities of yogurt and fermented cheese and yet have a high intolerance to American powdered milk.

Powdered yogurt and tablets have fewer bacteria per gram than well-prepared health food yogurt. These facts are supported by Soviet and German doctors.

So let's stop worrying about yogurt, but be discriminating in choosing the best we can find. You can, of course, make your own. There are many methods, but if you have not already found a successful one, you should find the following recipe acceptable.

Yogurt Recipe

1. Choose your own starter. It may be a commercial starter or some of your favorite yogurt, both available from health food stores.

2. Whether the milk is raw or pasteurized, heat it to just under the boiling point, being careful not to scorch it. Pasteurized milk has previously been heated only to 165° whereas boiling is 212°. In order to eliminate unfriendly bacteria, bring the milk almost to the boiling point. You may use a double boiler to heat the milk without fear of scorching. A thermometer is highly important for success.

3. Remove the milk from heat and allow to cool to between 90° and 110°. If you wish, you may add (or omit) 1 tablespoon powdered milk per pint of milk, and add 1 tablespoon of yogurt per pint of milk. (If you use

a commercial starter, follow the directions to the letter.) Stir the mixture gently.

4. Pour into individual jelly glasses or custard cups. Set them, up to the neck, in water in your covered electric frying pan and set the heat control so that it will not rise above 110°. Leave it, but watch it carefully toward the last, until the yogurt has just set. This usually takes between 8 and 12 hours. *Place containers in the refrigerator immediately*. Yogurt will continue to set further as it cools; if left too long in heat, it will become watery. After several days in the refrigerator it will become more acid, so use according to taste. Some people prefer less acid, some more. Many people do not like yogurt at first, but can cultivate a taste for it.

5. You may save the last container as a starter for the next batch, but in time, the culture will become weaker and you will have to buy new starter to ensure perfect yogurt.

References

1. *Science*. 16 June 1970.

2. Jose M. Rosell, M.D. "Yogurt and Kefir in Their Relationship to Health and Therapeutics." *Canadian Medical Association Journal*. Vol. 26, pp. 341-345, 1932.

3. Vincent Lucata. *Cultivating the Intestinal Flora for Better Health*. Santa Ana, Cal.: Continental Health Research (300 North Broadway, 92701).

4. Linda Clark. *Stay Young Longer*. New York, N.Y.: Pyramid Publications, 1968.

5. Ibid.

6. "Yogurt and Kefir."

7. *Cultivating the Intestinal Flora*.

8. Alexander Leaf, M.D. "Every Day Is a Gift When You Are Over 100." *National Geographic*. January 1973.

9. Ralph Pressman, Ph.D. "A Scientist Refutes Yogurt

Scare." *National Health Federation Bulletin.* January 1971.

10. *Archives of Ophthalmology.* 65, 181, 1961.
11. *Prevention.* November 1970.
12. "A Scientist Refutes Yogurt Scare."
13. *Prevention.* November 1970.
14. Linda Clark. *Natural Treatments for Common Ailments.* Old Greenwich, Conn.: Devin-Adair Co., 1976.

Will You Say
"Was It Really Worth It?"

IT WAS January 3rd. The bedside phone rang. Mrs. Clarence reached for another tissue before she answered it.

"Hullo," she croaked. "You probably can't understand a word I'm saying, because I have a turrible cold." She documented this understatement by sneezing loudly in a most unladylike manner.

It was just as well that the caller did not have phone-a-vision. Mrs. Clarence also looked "turrible." Her nose was red and streaming, her hair resembled dried straw, her skin was parched and her eyes had no more lustre than those of a statue.

"What's happened?" she said, echoing the question of her caller. "I guess it was just the holidays. I was late getting off my Christmas cards, late getting my Christmas shopping done, then I thought this year would be a good time to catch up with all our social obligations. You know," she reminded the caller, "you were at that wall-to-wall party we had, a party-to-end-all-parties—at least for a year.

"I made the mistake," she continued, "of sending out the invitations with my Christmas cards, and before I knew it, everybody else got the same idea. Back came invitations galore from others to try to pay back *their* social debts before the year ended. What a crush it turned out to be. And," she added, "the New Year's celebration didn't help any." After another violent

126

sneeze and a grab for more tissues, she decided to hang up.

Sound familiar? Holidays can just about make or break you, health-wise, at least for a while. Some of the reasons you know as well as I do. But there's one I'll wager you never thought of before.

The obvious reasons for the after-holiday letdown include too much tension, too much rush, too little rest. Just about everybody suddenly becomes "compulsive," as the psychologists call it; they feel they simply *must* cram all of the things they had put off for weeks into a short span of time. They also feel it necessary to keep up with the Joneses, and feel that Christmas wouldn't be Christmas without doing things the same old way, good or bad. But the real clincher (the one you hadn't thought of) is traditional *holiday eating.*

Holiday eating has probably contributed to the colds, to a good many pounds of overweight, to the deteriorated appearance of the Mrs. Clarences—and probably the Mr. Clarences, too. After the holidays are over, the honest ones will look in the mirror, assess their lack of well-being, and murmur, "Was it really worth it?"

Is there a way out? Of course.

I am going to leave the solutions to the obvious problems up to you. That is your department. You will have to figure out a new way to avoid the last-minute Christmas card binge. (Some people buy them on sale the previous January and address them in August.) Many form the habit of looking for the perfect gift for each person throughout the entire year, buying when it is available and less expensive—and when shopping can be done leisurely. I am only going to try to help you out of the holiday food trap. This is my department. Please give my suggestions a try for just one season. It should solve many of the disturbances and pressures developed in years past—and in a way which you never before understood.

What happens is this: with December comes cold weather. Houses become stuffy and overheated. Cold germs appear, and unless one is 100 percent well, rested and without tension, the cold can attack and flourish. Have you ever noticed that prior to December 15, few colds are in evidence? Then the parties begin! With the parties come sweets galore.

Do you know how germs are grown in a laboratory? *They are put in a sweet bath.* There they multiply. When you have been exposed to a germ and eat sweets, you become a walking laboratory—you and everybody else who is freeloading on traditional holiday treats: cookies, fruitcake and eggnog. Soon there are many walking laboratories who are culturing and multiplying and spreading germs. The coughs and the sniffles are in evidence everywhere. If you don't believe me, try counting the number of colds you see. You will soon run out of fingers and toes to add them up.

Christmas and the holiday season can be a pleasant time. People are loving, and giving, and mellow in thinking of others, perhaps more so than at any other time of year. This is good. We don't want to take the cheer out of Christmas. We merely want to escape the cheerlessness which follows when so many are sick, and cross and tired.

Most people are bound by tradition at Christmas, particularly traditional eating. They get out all their favorite cookie recipes, make fruitcake and order eggnog. Then, wanting to share these so-called delicacies, or show them off, or even get rid of them as the season drags to a close, they invite everyone they can think of to drop in. Nice custom. The trouble is that *everybody* serves the same fare. I sometimes think at this time of year that if I have to face one more piece of fruitcake or one more cup of eggnog, I can't stand it.

It is not really necessary to do the same thing in the same old way if there is a hazard involved. We no longer cook on wood stoves, use brooms to sweep our wall-to-wall carpeting, nor use a bar of soap to wash clothes. Why can't we find some new, healthful food ideas which better fit today's living; which pep us up instead of dragging us down?

There are substitutes for those germ-nurturing, pound-gaining, cavity-producing carbohydrates such as cookies and fruitcakes and the everlasting eggnog. (I, for one, am allergic to milk and raw eggs, and there are others like me.) Even dried fruits, including dates and figs, can be overdone. Such people as hypoglycemics (sufferers from low blood sugar) as well as diabetics cannot tolerate many natural sugars. Watch the coffee and alcohol, too. Yet if you serve such fare, what can these people (and their tribe is increasing) eat or drink at your house? You will render a public service if you will substitute healthful, delicious food and drink. You may even become famous. Guests will bless you.

Let me tell you of two people who learned their lesson, though they did not have to wait until the holidays to get the message. Since both are friends of mine, I can vouch that the stories are true.

Jean, a housewife and former model, suddenly realized that in spite of an excellent nutritional program, she was becoming more and more tired. She and her husband had recently built a new house and to save money were doing much of the finishing and painting themselves. Jean began upping her coffee intake to keep up her energy (so she thought), until she reached eight cups a day. Then she began to lean on her five o'clock cocktail to "relax" and get her through the preparation of the evening meal.

What really woke her up was what she saw in the mirror.

She decided to do away with the crutches of coffee and cocktails. She accomplished this by going on a few days of juices, plus vitamins and minerals and protein powders (added to water or juices). To her surprise her craving for both coffee and alcohol disappeared and her fatigue vanished with the restriction of both. I asked her what she used as substitutes. Instead of coffee, she drank hot bouillon. At a cocktail party, she drank water (everyone thought it was gin). She says that without coffee and alcohol, and with her good nutritional program, she now feels like a million.

Bob, a bachelor, had similar complaints. In addition to constant fatigue, though he was on an excellent nutritional program (he owns a health food store), he reported "sinking spells." He decided to analyze his eating and drinking just prior to these "attacks." By the process of elimination, he found that the offenders were sugar and coffee (in his case, instant coffee). He promptly gave up both with a vengeance. If a hostess serves him cake, or ice cream, or *anything* containing sugar, he refuses politely and firmly. And he spurns coffee. He says he has not had another one of those attacks of overpowering fatigue as long as he sticks to his guns, and though he had been subject to many colds each year, he has not had a single cold. But, if he backslides even once, his complaints return like a flash.

So change your holiday eating and see if you, too, don't reap rewards. If you are entertaining, don't get out all those traditional family heirloom recipes for cookies and candies and fruitcake. Make it simple. Substitute such things as hot, freshly popped corn (it is a whole grain and a nutritious food), raw nuts, salted soybeans (bought at a health food store or homemade) or hulled sunflower seeds. I find people can't stop eating them. And what a relief from all those sickening sweets!

For beverages, you can substitute bouillon on the rocks (with ice) or served hot, as they do on shipboard; or organic cider, also on the rocks with a twist of lemon, or served hot in a mug with a cinnamon stick as a stirrer. Or try a combination of half tomato juice and half orange juice which has been gently simmered with cinnamon sticks, a few cloves, and a pinch of nutmeg or mace. Serve that in a delicate cup, or thick mug, also with a cinnamon stick to stir. It is delicious! I serve it as a first course in the living room before every Thanksgiving and Christmas dinner and everyone asks for the recipe.

If you feel you must have a big "do," provide a gourmet buffet of delicious, healthful hors d'oeuvres. To find some unusual morsels that build you up instead of tearing you down, thumb your way through the cookbooks of Agnes Toms, Adelle Davis and Beatrice Trum Hunter, or others which you will find in the health food store. There are some *wonderful* ideas there, including the recipe for homemade salted soybeans.

So, dare to be different next season. You will find you can have your holidays and like them too. You can stay well and slim and attractive and need never again say on January 3rd after the holiday season is over, "Was it really worth it?"

Healthful Eating
in Cold Climates

I RECEIVED a letter from Ontario, Canada, which said:
"Many of us are frustrated by references in articles and
books to all the 'goodies' obtainable in the States, but
not here!

"In my area, the nearest health store is twenty miles
away. We live in a rural area but consider ourselves
fortunate that we *do* have access, albeit costly, to health
food stores. But how difficult it is in the land of long
winters to obtain fresh fruits and vegetables, let alone
organically grown ones! I do wish and pray you would
write an article for people in severe climates where all
our vegetables and fruits for many months are
'preserved' or trucked in a few thousand miles. I get the
impression that you writers live and think in terms of
California or Florida.

"As I write this, the wind is howling and blowing
snow to form even bigger snow dunes around our
house. Our view is fifteen miles—of deep snow. Even the
snow fences across the fields are hidden by the drifts. So,
please, can we have some hints on healthful eating
among the snow dunes?"

After reading this letter, I went around for several
days wringing my hands. What could I tell this woman—
and those like her, particularly when they are the rule,
not the exception?

After the hand-ringing stage had passed, I next began to follow my usual practice by sending out S.O.S.'s

to everyone who might suggest various ways to help. I sent an airmail letter to Beatrice Trum Hunter in New Hampshire (1). She and her husband live on a farm, so they, too, are usually snowbound in the winter.

Next, I called Paul Keene. He is the owner of Walnut Acres, at Penn's Creek, Pennsylvania, which grows organic grains, grinds and ships them, and other wonderful organic products, to homes and health food stores thousands of miles away. From these sources, plus a few of my own, I culled some help for you snowbounders which I hope will keep you healthy.

While it may be spring when many read this, and the worst of winter over, it couldn't be a better time to start to prepare for next winter. Use your phone, the new seed catalogues, a big notebook, and get busy.

First thing, the very fact that many of you live in rural areas gives you an advantage over city folks who can get to a store to get produce. You have *land!* How the city dwellers envy you! Even though you may have a short growing season, you can grow *something* to store throughout the winter which you can guarantee is organically grown. Apples, root vegetables such as potatoes, beets, carrots, turnips and onions, can be stored. They do not have to be canned or "preserved."

The more fragile foods such as peas, beans, corn, tomatoes, berries, peaches, apricots, cherries, etc., do not have to be canned, either. They can be frozen—the fruits raw, the vegetables with just a few seconds of blanching in boiling water and quick cooling in ice water. Enzymes, the body housecleaners, are killed by cooking but not by freezing. And, if they are not stored too long (like being carried over to next year), frozen fruits and vegetables retain more vitamin C and other nutrients than most canned foods.

A freezer will pay for itself many times over. I drop apricot halves, skin and all, and other large fruits cut into pieces, in containers or plastic bags in a mixture of water and a small amount of honey to taste, plus a small bit of ascorbic acid (vitamin C) to prevent browning or thawing. Berries and small fruits I lay on a cookie sheet without allowing them to touch each other, and freeze. When they are hard, I put them in a plastic bag and store them. You could also be lucky enough to find a farmer who raises organic meat or chickens, and buy in quantity at less price, for freezing.

If you cannot manage a garden alone, nor afford a freezer, by all means pick up that phone and start a co-operative gardening program, and join forces with some-one else who will help purchase a freezer. A new one, with a guarantee, from a mail order company is usually reasonably priced, particularly at sale time.

Scott Nearing, an ex-Vermonter now living in Maine, describes how they keep garden produce all winter (2). They store root crops in a cold cellar or root cellar. In bins or boxes, they place layers of leaves dropped from the trees in the fall, and put layers of vegetables—potatoes, carrots, celery root, beets, onions, turnips—in between generous layers of leaves. Mr. Nearing says that many of these vegetables last until the next July or August, and are crisp and firm. Apples stored in layers of dry sand kept until May and June. Cabbages hung upside down on strings, but not allowed to touch each other, kept until May. Some vegetables like broccoli, mustard greens, escarole, cos lettuce, celery, collards, kale, brussels sprouts, turnip greens and chard, are frostproof and can stay in the ground until they are covered with snow; thus they provide a variety before using up the root vegetables. Beans and peas can be dried, though I prefer to freeze them. Tomatoes I drop whole or cut up in the blender, add a dash of sea salt, put in a container and freeze raw instead of canning. For soups, juice, or cooking, they are easy to fix when needed.

But that is not all. Most winter-bound people become starved for raw greens for salads, and rightly so. Those who believe that 50 percent of our diet should be raw to assure best health need some help in this department. A kitchen garden and sprouts can help out here. Seed companies have curly-cress, which can be grown indoors in shallow trays on your kitchen window sill. It is ready to eat within ten days after planting and successive sowings should provide a continuous supply. It is excellent in salads, alone, or used with raw cabbage, celery, carrots, if you can't get lettuce, and perks up any sandwich. Parsley and chives can be grown indoors and are a help, too. Grated carrot, onion, cabbage, and green pepper (if you can find one) mixed with savory mayonnaise makes a delicious change from a green salad, and few people will turn down that Norwegian smorgasbord classic of grated carrot and raisins mixed with a sweeter type mayonnaise.

Catharyn Elwood is an expert on sprouts. Her book, *Feel Like A Million*, is loaded with ideas for choosing, growing and serving them (3). Equally informative is *Add a Few Sprouts* by Martha Oliver(4). Although the choice of seeds to sprout is endless, most people prefer mung beans (you can float away the hulls in a bowl of water after sprouting), alfalfa, and wheat seed. These sprouts are literally packed with vitamins. The seeds can be stored the year around and then, after sprouting, be added to salads, sandwiches, or dropped at the last minute into omelets or soups to heat through only, not cook. Remember that it is raw food you are looking for. There are more enzymes and nutrients in raw sprouts than cooked. Both books will give you much valuable sprout information. (For my method of sprouting see "Special Preparation Methods" in "The Issue Is Survival.")

Another delicious addition to salads is *raw* Jerusalem

artichokes, sliced thin. Once you start them in your garden, even in a flower bed (they grow tall), they spread. You dig up the roots in the fall like potatoes and they can keep for ages in a refrigerator or root cellar. They are nutritious, taste like Chinese water chestnuts, and are truly delicious.

Don't forget about nuts! They, too, are raw and protected by shells to keep fresh for a whole year, to eat straight from the shell or in food mixtures. Sunflower seeds are another raw bonus. To keep indefinitely, buy them in vacuum-packed tins, already shelled. They make a wonderful mid-meal snack for children and adults alike. A few will give you a quick pickup in energy and are a good source of protein and vitamins.

One of the happiest finds for nutritious eating, year-round, is the fourteen-grain cereal suggested by Dr. William D. Kelley, of Texas. Although it is intended as a cereal, it could be eaten at other meals. You buy a package of each of the following: wheat berries, buckwheat, rye, barley, oat groats, millet, sesame seeds, lentils, brown rice, flax, corn (or popcorn), alfalfa seeds, mung beans, and almonds. Mix the fourteen ingredients in a large container, or take smaller equal parts of each and combine in a quart jar, keeping the remainder refrigerated or in a very cool place. Each night take three or four tablespoons of this mixture per person and grind it in a sturdy blender or electric seed mill. Cover with water and allow to stand overnight at room temperature. In the morning, add fruit, a dribble of raw honey, milk, cream or soy milk (reconstituted from soy powder from health stores). This cereal is *always* supposed to be eaten raw. It is inexpensive per serving and if kept cool, an excellent keeper. Mixed with diced or shredded apple during the winter, and other fruits as they come into season, Dr. Kelley says it is extremely rich in nutrients and an excellent body builder.

Warning: Most of these seeds are available from health stores. If you get some of them from a feed store, *be sure* they have not been treated with deadly chemicals!

These ideas, plus others you will no doubt collect as you go along, can provide a foundation for healthful eating in any climate. In addition, you can work out a co-op plan to have shipped to you some fresh organic food and citrus fruits. Also, find a farmer who supplies fertile eggs. Bake your own bread weekly. If you drink milk, look for a safe source of tested raw milk and dairy products in your rural community. By combining all these wonderful foods, you can be as healthy or healthier than the rest of us. In fact, with such healthful, delicious fare, we would like to be snowed in with you!

References

1. Beatrice Trum Hunter. *The Natural Foods Cookbook.* New York, N.Y.: Pyramid Publications, 1967.

2. Scott Nearing. *Living the Good Life.* New York, N.Y.: Schocken Books, 1972.

3. Catharyn Elwood. *Feel Like a Million.* New York, N.Y.: Pocket Books, 1968.

4. Martha Oliver. *Add a Few Sprouts.* New Canaan, Conn.: Keats Publishing, 1975.

Have You Tried Clay?

JUST AS many of us had decided nothing new was ever going to happen in the health field, a new and exciting breakthrough has occurred. Those who have had an advance peek at this new therapy, the use of clay, are all a'quiver. Used externally and internally, the results are almost unbelievable. Yet, having tried it myself and watched others who are using it, there is no doubt that clay has vast potential for improving health.

Clay has, apparently, been used for centuries in Europe but most of us had not known about it since it was practically unheard of in the United States. It took a book, recently published, to wake us up to its tremendous healing possibilities. The book, *Our Earth, Our Cure*, written by Raymond Dextreit and translated into English by Michel Abehsera, appeared in late 1974 in a large, flat, handsome paperback. The second printing of the book was sold out within one-and-a-half months. It is the composite of forty-three books, written by Raymond Dextreit, who has had thirty-two years of practice and experience in working with clay as well as with herbs and natural foods. The information in the book about herbs and foods is excellent, but the explanation of clay, and what it can do for you, came as an electric shock. It tells what clay to use, where to get it and how to use it. The treatment is a simple, do-it-yourself technique to be used in any home, and the cost, compared to drugs and medication, is negligible (1).

I first heard about clay more than four years ago. A man wrote me that on his property in the mountains of a lightly populated state he had made an unusual discovery. A trapper noticed that several kinds of animals —elk, deer, coyote, and lynx—were congregating in a certain area which contained an unusual deposit of clay. Apparently they were licking it or, if injured, rolling in it to obtain relief from their injuries or ailments. The trapper took some of this clay to the landowner to see if he could find out what was in it that attracted animals to it. The owner had it analyzed by a laboratory and the secret, which I will describe later, was discovered.

Mr. Dextreit tells us that animals seem to know instinctively the help that clay—often in the form of mud—can provide them when they are ill or wounded. He reports that horses have been cured of hoof gangrene, cows of hoof and mouth disease. Veterinarians in this country who have tried it are also impressed with clay. They have used it on domestic animals and pets, often with spectacular results. The clay is used on animals as it can be used on humans—in paste form on the skin, or added to drinking water. After hearing of friends who put clay in the bottom of the water dish of their dogs, and noting that even old, sedate dogs began to caper about with renewed vitality, I tried it on my two cats. One of them, who is generally uncooperative, refused to taste the clay water, but the other, once he started drinking it, couldn't stop. Several days later he began to cavort like a kitten, although he is four years old.

Veterinarians supply other findings. One cat brought in to be put to sleep because of an accidental amputation of its tail by a lawn mower, which had caused gangrene, was instead treated externally with the clay and the gangrene completely and quickly healed. Clay was also used to treat osteomyelitis in horses by one veterinarian, while another injected a thin solution of clay and water into a calf with terminal pneumonia. Within eight hours, the secretions of mucus and other symptoms had disappeared.

External Results

What about people? The following reports have been contributed by doctors and laymen. First let's look at the effects of clay used externally.

One doctor testified that clay was the only remedy found to heal fiddleback spider bites, common in the area where the doctor practices. This doctor also stated that clay was the best treatment for burns yet noted, and that varicose ulcers responded to clay treatment, even in one patient who had been afflicted for seventeen years. In all cases, the clay was applied externally.

Another doctor told me that the clay applied to acne and other skin problems has been so successful that he could not keep it in stock for his patients. He also uses it successfully for contact dermatitis and for resistant rashes, which he believes are the result of the body's elimination of toxins through the skin. If so, clay taken internally also seems to be indicated. This doctor started using clay long before *Our Earth, Our Cure* was published, when he had read that Mahatma Gandhi used clay in the form of mud poultices (2).

Other reports of external use of clay include:

- A wet pack or poultice applied daily to a boil brought it to a head in three days, and the culture of the wound was found to be sterile.
- Eczema, treated by "everything" for ten years, was cleared from hands in two days.
- Bee stings and insect stings respond promptly.
- A poultice applied to corns and calluses both on and between the toes and left for three days, then renewed for three more days, caused the afflictions to disappear.
- Hemorrhoids have been alleviated.

- Ringworm was cleared by repeated application of a clay-and-water solution.
- Pinkeye was cleared in one-and-a-half days.
- Doctors and patients alike are enthusiastic about the use of clay packs on the face. It has cleared up pimples, and because it leaves the skin smooth, soft and younger looking, it is used widely as a cosmetic. Because it is somewhat drying, one doctor recommends that his patients use olive oil after removing the clay mask from the face.
- A teenage boy received a leg scratch; it resisted medical treatment and the leg developed gangrene. The doctor's verdict: amputation! However, the boy's father, who refused the amputation and had heard about the clay, applied it on his son's leg and in a few days the gangrene disappeared and the leg was saved. Today, years later, the leg is as good as new, with the exception of scars.
- One woman had a chronic sore on her face which had long refused to heal. She tried the clay, which cleared the sore within two days.
- Laboratory tests show that clay can combat staph germs.

The reports cited thus far have been collected from sources other than those mentioned in the book, *Our Earth, Our Cure.* You will find additional reports there.

Internal Use of Clay

The use of clay internally is even more incredible. We have long heard of people eating clay, a practice known as *pica*. The dictionary defines pica as follows: *depraved or perverted appetite or craving for unnatural food, as chalk, clay, etc., common in chlorosis (iron deficiency), pregnancy, etc.*

This craving may not be 'depraved or perverted at all, but makes sense when you know what clay contains. I have the laboratory analyses of three clays before me, and the mineral content, particularly of calcium, iron and silica plus the trace minerals (those appearing in small amounts) is impressive. On reading these analyses, it instantly becomes clear why these people, as well as animals, have an appetite for clay. They are merely craving minerals in which they are deficient. It also explains why Raymond Dextreit states that taking clay internally every day has reversed anemia within one month. The clay supplies iron in an organic, easily assimilated form.

Gandhi reports (3) that clean earth may be eaten in order to overcome constipation. As a matter of fact, this is the first benefit noted by most people who begin taking the clay internally; their elimination improves.

Clay can be taken mixed with water in the form of paste. A friend of mine was afflicted with amoebic dysentery when she lived in a European country as a small child. Since nothing else helped, the doctors finally prescribed one teaspoon of regular, common tea, every hour, and nothing else. For a five-year-old child, this was a stringent treatment, but the doctors were trying to "starve" the amoeba, they insisted. When the mother realized that they were also starving her child, she dismissed the doctors and took matters into her own hands. She spoon-fed moistened clay to her daughter and within a short time the amoeba had completely disappeared. Raymond Dextreit states that clay removes parasites and worms from the intestinal tract, and a doctor in this country, whom I interviewed, confirms it.

Mr. Dextreit suggests an easy way to take clay internally, regardless of the disturbance you wish to treat. He says to put one teaspoon of the dry powdered clay (source listed later) in the bottom of a glass. Add half a glass of unboiled water, stir well, but remove the metal spoon and let the mixture sit overnight. In the morning, on an empty stomach fifteen to twenty minutes before breakfast, drink the liquid. You may stir it once again, remixing the clay and water, since it will settle during the night leaving a clear liquid, or you may take the clear liquid only, without stirring the mixture. Mr. Dextreit states that people who drink the clear liquid seem to get as good results as those who remix the clay with the water.

Some find that they get even better results by drinking the clay mixture or clay water at bedtime. Since the clay absorbs, or draws out, poisons from the intestines, I became a little worried for fear it might also remove vitamins from the intestinal tract. I wrote to the publisher, who wrote to Mr. Dextreit in Europe. He answered the question by saying that the clay does not destroy vitamins; it actually enhances or expands their potency.

What else has been accomplished by clay used internally?

- In one case, putting the clay powder into double 00 (00) size capsules and taking two, four times daily, removed all symptoms of an internal ulcer within seven days.
- Dr. Meyer-Camberg, of Europe, recommends the mineral-rich clay for many different purposes. One is to neutralize poisons. If arsenic or some other poison is accidentally swallowed, he recommends immediately taking one teaspoonful of clay mixed in water, and then another teaspoonful every hour for six hours. Evidently the clay binds the toxic poisons and nullifies them, leaving no harmful effects upon the body.
- Case after case provides testimony that clay cleanses the bloodstream. Dextreit states that

clay will enrich the blood as well as cleanse it. He says, "The same teaspoon of clay can cure an obstinate carbuncle and a tenacious anemia ... in a month you can expect an impressive increase of red blood cells." He adds something even more incredible: "Clay does more than restore a particular substance lacking in the body. ... It stimulates the deficient organ and helps the restoration of the failing function."

He adds, "In cases of organic disorders, its intense activity eliminates and destroys unhealthy cells and activates the rebuilding of healthy ones. . . . It not only cures diarrhea and constipation, it acts on all of the organs—on the whole organism."

There is more, much more, about clay in the book *Our Earth, Our Cure,* that you cannot afford to miss. Don't expect some of these transformations to appear overnight. Some conditions may disappear more quickly than others, whereas other effects such as glandular and organ stimulation may take more time and the results are more subtle. You will need to experiment and keep trying, but keep up the treatment until you learn for yourself what clay can do.

Which Clay?

What type of clay should you use? There are many types of clay in different parts of the world.

According to *Here's Health* magazine, an English publication, various clays (often in the form of mud) are used by spas the world over for relieving chronic conditions. *Here's Health* writes, "There is nothing like mud for cleansing the blood. Ordinary garden mud would not do much to improve your complexion, but specially located muds have been found to have a cleansing and purifying effect on the skin.

"Adeko Mud comes from the Moroccan mountains

and contains minerals. This mud comes in dry form and when water is added can be used as a shampoo, a face mask, or a body wash. The product is imported to Britain by a Danish Company.

"From the other side of the world comes a fossilized earth from a special quarry in Ireland. A third company makes clay and mud products which originate in the Dead Sea and also contain minerals." (4) (These clays are not available in the United States.)

In *Our Earth, Our Cure*, Raymond Dextreit mentions a fine-textured green clay that he finds in France, and particularly recommends for internal use. (Its source in the United States is given in the shopping guide at the end of the book.) Mr. Dextreit states that even ordinary potter's clay can be beneficial but I, personally, tend to lean toward the clays which have been tested and found to contain minerals. I find that certain clays are better for certain purposes: some for external use, some for internal use. Because of their individuality as well as the different needs of individual people, you may wish to try several until you choose the one you prefer. I keep four kinds on hand and use them for various purposes.

One company imports not only the green clay mentioned by Mr. Dextreit, but also excellent clay cosmetics as well as a toothpaste which combines the clay, sea salt and anise flavoring. The prices of these products are surprisingly inexpensive as compared with costs of other cosmetics.

The green clay is available at The Three Sheaves, 16 Hudson Street, New York, N.Y. 10013, if unavailable at your health store.

References

1. Raymond Dextreit. *Our Earth, Our Cure*. Translated by Michel Abehsera. Brooklyn, N.Y.: Swan House Publishing Co. (P.O. Box 170, 11223), 1974.

2. M. K. Gandhi. *Key to Health*. Ahmedabad, India: Navajivan Press.
3. Ibid.
4. *Here's Health*, January 1975.

How to Feel Better within Days

LESS THAN a week ago, I woke up one morning feeling blah. There is no other adequate description of the way I felt; I just felt blah! I was dragging, my energy level was low, and I felt as if I had had it!

This morning I woke up feeling marvelous, on top of the world, with energy to spare and that good-to-be-alive feeling. I made this change within a single week, and all by myself. You can do the same thing.

It happens to us all, no matter how healthy. As a matter of fact, Dr. Bernard Jensen, who has treated thousands of patients by natural methods, says that he has never seen a completely healthy person(1). On top of this, we eat, drink and breathe the wrong things, become tense (which interferes with smooth body function) and perhaps we get too little regular exercise. The result: our digestions slow down, our bodies become choked with poisons, we become tired and feel miserable. Dr. Jensen says, "A tired body cannot eliminate, absorb, digest, plan, love or concentrate properly."

So what to do? Filling up on drugs merely makes matters worse. Drugs, unless used for emergency lifesaving purposes, merely mask symptoms but do not remove them. In fact, many poisons stored in the body may be caused by drugs. I recall reading many years ago that during a detoxification diet, or a colonic (I don't remember which), a natural doctor found the body of one of

147

his patients ejecting drugs which had been taken over forty years previously!

Going to a hospital for a rest cure is no good, since the poor hospital diet, plus the drugs they insist upon giving people, only make matters worse. Happily, there is something exciting happening in England, where a fringe-medicine hospital has been planned. It will provide such unorthodox medical treatments as homeopathy, acupuncture, osteopathy, nature cures, and even faith healing. The hospital will have five sections. It will have an education center for *doctors* to learn nutrition and unorthodox medicine. It will have a surgical wing for necessary surgery only. It will have a maternity wing for natural childbirth, as well as for education of mothers both before and after pregnancy. It will have a medical wing for chronically ill people suffering from asthma, bronchitis, cancer, diabetes, heart conditions, and so forth, with curative treatments taught for home use afterwards. Finally, there will be a chapel and meditation center for people of all religions. Music and color therapy will also be available here(2). Three cheers for England! The United States should have one in every city; they would be swamped.

A third possibility for people who merely need a tune-up (as I did) would be a spa where you are both pampered and treated by natural methods(3). This is a lovely idea, but not practical for me. I cannot leave my work responsibilities, home, or garden, in these days of hard-to-find help and property vandalism. So, since a spa was not in the cards for me, I had to figure out my own plan. I did and it worked. Here is how.

To begin with, I work hard, long hours. Dr. Jensen tells us that a rested body is the one which gets well. Many times overwork is the cause of physical problems. Getting away from it all may help some, but if you are still tense, you are defeating yourself, he says. So he advises letting go, mentally *and* physically, and letting recuperation take place(4).

This I did. I finished up the most demanding deadlines, put my desk in order, the cover on my typewriter and shut the door to my office. I decided I would take four days—four blissful days—of doing only what I felt like doing, nothing I was supposed to do. I love my home, which is located in a healthful climate, but which I seldom have time to notice. The air is good, but I seldom take time to breathe it. I realized that I had everything I needed right where I was, and also where I was the most comfortable. But even if I had lived in an apartment in a city, I could have done most of the same things. It isn't where you are, but what you are doing there, I decided, which is important.

I chose light reading instead of heavy educational literature. I got out some knitting, not because I like it, but because it is relaxing and gives my mind a rest. I was then ready for the next step: a detoxification diet. I bought all the necessary supplies and was ready to go. I didn't even tell anyone I was going to follow this four-day program. Otherwise, friends would have tried to talk me out of it (as they often do a would-be reducer) or might even call in alarm at regular intervals to see how I was. I merely told my family I was going to rest for a few days, to which they said, "Hurray!"

You may know by this time, from reading my various books and articles, that I do not believe in complete fasting. I, and a growing number of therapists, consider fasting (with no foods and water only) extremely dangerous. We are not living in biblical days, but in a polluted world. Our bodies, scientists tell us, are loaded with pesticides and other poisons from food, water and air. If we start to fast on water these poisons are released too quickly into the bloodstream and can cause self-poisoning, and severe illness in many cases.

So I did it the safe way: with cleansing juices, and a little fruit now and then, to slow down the poison excretion and dilute the effect on the body. Since detoxification takes place through the intestines, the lungs, the kidneys, and the skin, I helped these processes by getting a little sun on my skin every day, breathing deeply outdoors and sleeping as long as possible, including a daily nap. I also took a long, warm tub soak, daily. You can exercise or walk, although I didn't.

The cleansing dietary program I used is one I have used before and swear by. The first time I heard of it was from an assistant to the originator of the program, Stanley A. Burroughs, who has since left this country (I wish I knew where he is, to thank him). The assistant wrote to tell me of a patient who was bedridden with all sorts of minor ailments and was promised that the Burroughs program would bring miracles as well as get the patient out of bed in ten days. It did. I didn't believe it until I tried it myself, and since then I have mentioned it to numerous other people, all of whom agree that they, too, end up feeling absolutely wonderful. This program, which Mr. Burroughs calls the Master Cleanser, is designed to:

- dissolve toxins and mucus throughout the body
- cleanse the kidneys and the digestive system
- purify glands and cells
- eliminate all unusable waste and hardened material in the joints and muscles
- relieve pressure and irritation in nerves, arteries and blood vessels
- build a healthy bloodstream

Mr. Burroughs also states that using this program three or four times a year will do wonders for less serious or mild conditions, or can be used more often for more serious conditions. He recommends, as an average, sticking to it for ten days. As you know by now, I used it for only four days. But the results were remarkable for me. Others will have to decide for themselves how long to continue. I believe there is no point in letting yourself get weak; in fact, I would be inclined to think that *great* weakness might be a warning to STOP, or to continue only under a doctor's supervision.

The Program
(as outlined by Mr. Burroughs)

Combine the juice of ½ lemon with two tablespoons of a certain type of sweetening, and add to an 8 ounce glass of hot water. The sweeteners are a *must*, according to Mr. Burroughs, to balance the lemon and achieve desired results. The only sweetenings allowed are any kind of unsulphured molasses: Grandma's, Barbados, Louisiana, or blackstrap. Some people who have trouble with these since they are slightly laxative (though usually a good thing in a cleansing program), use pure maple syrup with Mr. Burroughs' blessing. He does not condone honey for this program.

You are to drink this concoction, he says, from 6 to 12 times a day, whenever you feel hungry. *Be sure to use a straw*. Both lemon juice and molasses, if left on the teeth, can erode enamel. In any case, rinse your mouth with clear water after taking, just to be sure. Take no other food during the full time of the diet.

Most people use the mixture about six times daily. If you are not eliminating properly, Mr. Burroughs suggests a herb laxative tea, available at health food stores.

Mr. Burroughs assures us that there is no danger in this program; the only thing you can lose, he says, is mucus, waste and disease. He says healthy tissue is not affected. But he warns *not* to vary the amount of lemon juice per glass.

Now I must confess that I cheated. I had just read

that watermelon is a marvelous diuretic, so I rewarded myself each afternoon with a small serving of watermelon. And since the repetition is boring, I took some brewer's yeast in water or broth at noontime or alternated the lemon-juice drinks with tomato juice or some fresh, natural vegetable juice. I also took plenty of vitamin C to speed neutralization of any poisons, even though Mr. Burroughs does not approve of supplements taken during this cleansing program. (Sorry about that, Mr. Burroughs.) After all, blackstrap, which was my choice of sweetening, is loaded with natural iron, calcium, potassium, and B vitamins. Lemon juice also contains vitamin C.

Now what do you do *after* you have decided to stop this program? Mr. Burroughs' suggestions are: eat, as often as you are hungry, a soup made of fresh vegetables, or using brown rice. He believes that you should continue to drink liquids freely for two days after coming off the diet and take no meat, eggs, fish, breads, pastries, etc. On the third day he believes normal eating can be resumed. Coming off the program is crucial!

Meanwhile, now is the time to improve your overall diet. There is no point in going back to the old junk which helped to get you into the condition you have just tried to correct. This diet is a marvelous opportunity to get rid of some of your addictions. Where other people may become addicted to sugar or alcohol, I am a pushover for all of the good natural breads available in California. This is an easy way to acquire a spare tire. I have lost a bread addiction whenever I have followed this diet, a great benefit for me.

Other good things have happened to me, too. Although you may look a little seamy when you first get off the diet, this will change, since you will be feeling so good you can't help but look better soon. I also lose weight on the diet (some of it returns, but less if I give up that old bogey-for-me, bread). Other little nagging things disappear. I won't enumerate them since yours may differ from mine. What does apply to everyone I have watched on this diet, is that they all report they feel like a million dollars and usually soon look the part, too.

What I never can understand is why I don't do this oftener. It is such a quick and rewarding program, even for prevention purposes, without waiting until you feel miserable. So help me, from now on, I am going to repeat it three times a year.

Meanwhile, here is a salute to Stanley A. Burroughs, wherever you are, for originating the Master Cleanser. It really works. Thank you.

References

1. Dr. Bernard Jensen. *World Keys to Health and Longevity*. Escondido, Cal.: Omni Publishers, 1975.

2. *Here's Health* (English magazine). May 1975.

3. Robert and Raye Yaller. *The Health Spas: World Guidebook to Health Spas, Mineral Baths and Nature Cure Centers*. Santa Barbara, Cal.: Woodbridge Press Publishing Co., 1975.

4. *World Keys to Health and Longevity*.

Vegetarians, Beware!

I HAVE received a letter from the director of a Zen Center in a large city in California. The letter is both provocative and intelligent. It reads:

Dear Linda:
I am writing you on behalf of Zen Center, thinking you would possibly be willing to help us consider what kind of vegetarian diet our groups should choose and follow.

We are not strict vegetarians. Within our communities we do not eat any meat, though we do eat cheese, eggs, milk. When eating out at restaurants or friends' homes, we eat what is served, including meat. So, primarily, on a day-to-day basis, we are vegetarians. Some of us, however, have been eating almost entirely Zen Center food for eight years now, which consists of organically raised food, and, when possible, we grow our own food, produce our own eggs and make our own bread.

Our diet has kept changing, influenced more or less by current fads: macrobiotic, mucusless, Essene gospel, and others, now protein. We would like to develop a diet unsusceptible to fads, one which people can live on, not just for a few months, but for a lifetime. We have children in some of our groups, so they must be considered too. We are interested in any research you have found on vegetarianism. Our feeling is that one week or one month is not much of a test. Often problems do not show up for five, ten, fifty years. Though we admit to being guinea pigs, we like to do the best we can.

Vegetarianism seems to be largely an unexplored area, or explored only by those on some fad trip. Some people may like it, but it would not do to impose it on everybody.

Thank you for any help you can give us. Sincerely, E.B.

Dear E.B.: It is a joy to answer a letter so intelligent and open minded. Many vegetarians are on the defensive, as fiercely protective about their choice of diet as they are about their politics or religion, as if these choices were the *only* acceptable solutions. Yet what may help one, in any area of life, may not necessarily help another. Also, nutritionally speaking, what one eats occasionally does not make or break good health. It is what one eats day in and day out, that is important in the long run. So your permissive attitude when eating out is commendable.

I will gladly share with you the results of the research I have found on the subject, showing both sides. From this information, I believe a pattern will emerge so that each person can work out his own diet to produce the best health for him, since ultimately, everyone wants to be healthy.

Why Do People Become Vegetarians?

Some people choose vegetarianism because of religious beliefs. Others claim they cannot bear to hurt animals. (One cannot always use kindness to animals as the only reason, since recent publications show that plants have feelings, too (1).) The history of civilization shows that our diet has for many centuries been based on survival of the fittest. Birds eat worms, as well as seeds. Big fish eat smaller fish. Man, who originally was carnivorous, gradually became omnivorous, adding herbs, seeds and nuts, but still retaining flesh foods in his diet. He caught his prey, whether animal or fish, and ate it, not so much by choice, but to survive. Otherwise you and I would not be here now. That food was built into our genes, making us what we are today. The genes of various races differ, partly because of different geographical locations with different diets.

In time, the genes of all races adapt to each others' foods. But the body does not like sudden change; it takes time to adjust to any new diet. This applies to vegetarianism, too.

I love animals. I also love plants. But I also want to be healthy, as you do. The time may come in future centuries when we will not eat flesh foods because our bodies, and those of our successors will have *gradually* changed to adapt to different food. We could not suddenly move to Mars without having problems with weightlessness, temperature change and a completely strange diet. We would have to learn to adapt first. So it may not be healthy or even safe to decide today to become a vegetarian tomorrow.

Vegetarianism is, as you say, spreading like a fad. It is showing up in the proliferating vegetarian restaurants, on college campuses, and is being adopted by a growing number of celebrities. This adds status to the movement. Many people are influencing others, especially the younger generation, who are among those, as you say, on a fad trip. They are making the choice emotionally, not intelligently. We should not choose anything so important to health just because "everyone else is doing it." (This tendency also applies to the drug invasion, and has caused some sobering, sad results.) Physically, we are all as different as our finger prints. Vegetarianism, if chosen, should be based on *your* body, *your* needs. You are a law unto yourself and even members of the same family or community may not thrive on exactly the same diet.

Some people have decided upon vegetarianism because flesh foods are so expensive. If so, there are less expensive alternatives. Protein foods are less expensive than medical bills. Others claim that meat is contaminated with chemicals and hormones, but then, so are plants, usually being sprinkled with pesticides. If you really want safer foods of any kind, you can find them, though it takes effort.

Why Is Protein So Important?

We are all largely made of protein. Researchers galore have discovered this undeniable fact. The United States Yearbook of Agriculture, 1939 (far ahead of its time nutritionally) states that protein may be the "secret of life." Consider these facts: (2)

- Muscles (including your heart) are made of protein.
- Glands and organs are made of protein. This includes liver, kidneys, even your eyes.
- Hair and skin are almost 98 percent protein.
- Secretions of various glands are made of protein: thyroxin (from thyroid), pancreatin (from the pancreas), secretions from the pituitary, a master gland which regulates your size and other functions, and many, many more, are *all made of protein.*

Prolonged protein deficiency can cause:

anemia
liver disease
peptic ulcer

kidney disease
poor resistance to infection; poor wound healing
and body repair
irritability
fatigue and lack of energy; weakness
wasting tissues
higher cholesterol
poor circulation
constipation
edema (water storage causing overweight)
early aging
and many others.

Dr. Valmiri Ramalingaswami, an Indian researcher, states that since a shortage of protein affects the entire body adversely, protein must be supplied regularly, on a daily basis, to replace that constantly used up by body activities. Otherwise, one organ will borrow from another, until the whole body collapses. This Indian doctor knows whereof he speaks. As Dr. Bernard Jensen says, "In India people live to the average age of thirty-one or thirty-two years, and it is caused by a lack of protein. Eighty percent of their diet is lacking in protein."(3)

Adelle Davis hit the nail right on the head when she said, "Since your body structure is largely protein, an undersupply can bring about aging with depressing speed. . . . Muscles lose tone; wrinkles appear; aging creeps on; and you, my dear, are going to pot." (4) (Not the kind you smoke.)

Delayed reactions to vegetarianism, as you state in your letter, may not show up for five, ten, fifty years. You are so right. Sometimes they do not show up until the next generation. For proof, witness the following diet study. In the 1940s Francis F. Pottenger Jr., M.D., conducted a study (complete with colored movies) of 900 cats divided into two groups. One group was fed raw protein, raw milk. These cats remained healthy and produced healthy kittens, generation after generation. The second group was fed the type of diet which, for them, paralleled our human diet: cooked food and pasteurized milk. This group developed ailments exactly like humans:

    diarrhea
    pneumonia
    heart trouble
    kidney disease
    thyroid trouble
    paralysis
    diminished sex interest
    and many others.

It sometimes took three generations of kittens on this diet to produce these ailments, but eventually they appeared. The second generation was less healthy than the first generation. The third generation was still weaker, and the cats were far worse specimens of health (5). So do not underestimate that delayed reaction of vegetarianism.

I can hear readers impatiently saying, "O.K., O.K., Let's get on with it. Agreed that we need protein, does this mean we must have animal protein? Aren't there safe alternatives?" Certainly there are other kinds of proteins. Let's see what they are and what researchers have learned about them.

Protein Alternatives

Proteins are made up of factors called amino acids. Some proteins are complete proteins, able to supply the body requirements adequately. Other proteins are incomplete. There are approximately twenty-two amino acids in all, twelve of which can be manufactured from other materials by the body. But eight to ten of the amino acids, called "essential," annot be manufactured and can only be supplied by foods, such as the complete proteins. Most animal protein contains all of these essen·

159

tial amino acids, and together with a few other foods to be mentioned later, are complete proteins.

Vegetable proteins lack—except, perhaps, for soybeans—one or more of these essential acids, thus are termed "incomplete" proteins. They do not protect the body as complete proteins do. Tests show that if a missing amino acid is supplied at *a different time* from the other essential amino acids, the body cannot use it. Eating it later in the day will not suffice; it must be *combined with* the other essential amino acids *at the same meal.*

It is true that certain tribes have thrived on vegetarian diets of seeds, grains, plants, nuts, sprouts, and so on, but these tribes may have unwittingly learned to combine certain foods to produce a complete protein formula.

Many vegetarians will argue that horses, cows and other animals are well and strong, yet do not eat flesh foods. True. I checked this with a veterinarian who said that the digestive systems of these animals are totally different from human digestive systems and can manufacture different enzymes which man cannot. These animals belong to the grass-eating group. Other animals belong to the flesh-eating group. Man can eat both types of food. So man's need cannot always be gauged by animal criteria and vice versa. But there is a far more important problem for man to understand in connection with vegetarianism.

Man needs vitamin B-12 in order to be strong and healthy. B-12 is one of the hardest vitamins not only to get, but to assimilate. What happens when you do not get enough B-12? Plenty. A deficiency of this vitamin can cause anemia, either simple or pernicious. Oded Abramsky, M.D., Department of Neurology, Hadassah University, Jerusalem, warns that as a result of B-12 deficiency, the following changes in the nervous system may occur: weakness, soreness in legs and arms; diminished reflex response and sensory perception; difficulty in walking and eventually in speaking; possible jerking of limbs plus a gradual disintegration of the spinal and nervous systems. *These symptoms may not became apparent until it is too late* (that delayed reaction again), at which time permanent mental deterioration as well as physical paralysis may occur. What is little known is that a B-12 deficiency may also cause a type of brain damage resembling schizophrenia.

If you are already a vegetarian and have noticed sore mouth, stiffness, a feeling of numbness, shooting pains or a pins-and-needles sensation as well as hot-and-cold sensations (or any of the other symptoms mentioned above), run, don't walk, to the nearest doctor for a series of B-12 injections. One study has shown that the amount of B-12 is lower in vegetarians than in non-vegetarians because *plants contain little or no* B-12. Animal protein is almost the only reliable and sufficient source of this vitamin. Eggs, and dairy products, as well as flesh foods contain it in sufficient amounts to prevent pernicious anemia and resulting nerve damage. Once contracted, the ailment usually cannot be reversed by food, but by injections only. The richest source of B-12 is liver (it takes tons of liver to yield a few crystals of B-12) and liver is the basis for B-12 injections. George Bernard Shaw, the famous long-time vegetarian, called the liver he was finally forced to take, his "medicine."

In addition to dairy products and eggs, as well as meat, fish and fowl, a few vegetable sources such as peanuts, seaweed, Concord grapes and soybeans contain some B-12. Some brewer's yeast contains it only if bred to include it, a recent improvement, and will state on the label if it is present. Wheat germ contains some B-12, but raw soybeans are deficient in B-12 and create a still greater need for it. If you were to take B-12 in supplement form, you probably would not assimilate it, since it is notoriously difficult to assimilate straight from the bottle. Also, to my knowledge, no one knows how much is needed, partly because of individual differences.

As for amino acids, it is possible to combine certain incomplete proteins, which are short in one amino acid, with other incomplete proteins, which are short in another. Frances Moore Lappé has provided how-to help in her excellent little book *Diet for a Small Planet* (6). Many vegetarians are already using this book to produce "completed" proteins from combinations of incomplete ones. Ray Wolf, writing in *Organic Gardening* (7), says, "Without all the essential amino acids (those which your body cannot produce), your body cannot turn food into energy. If only one amino acid is missing, the system won't work. . . . According to Frances Moore Lappé, whole wheat is deficient in two amino acids, rye in three, egg noodles in two, bulgur in two, barley in two, brown rice in two, oatmeal in two, and millet in one."

But even completed plant proteins do not guarantee B-12, which is another problem entirely. However, by adding any of the animal proteins to the above proteins, you are safe. Eventually we may learn about more plant foods which are complete proteins within themselves or which contain B-12, but until then, Carlton Fredericks. Ph.D, states that some animal protein is *needed at each meal.*

Do You Digest It?

A *New York Times* article (8) stated, "What attracts many people to vegetarianism is [their] poor health. We call these 'stomach vegetarians.' As soon as they become well again, they turn back to eating meat." Some people who change over to vegetarianism insist that they immediately feel better, which is probably true. In fact, the reason for this may be the spark that triggers someone over to vegetarianism in the first place. Here is why:

Protein of any kind, especially flesh food, *cannot be digested without sufficient stomach acid* known as hydrochloric acid, or HCl. Undigested protein can produce toxins which result from fermented undigested food, causing gas and other symptoms of indigestion. If a person is deficient in HCl, which is common, and turns to vegetarianism, the indigestion problems seem to disappear. HCl is not now as necessary, yet the longer vegetarianism continues, the less HCl the body manufactures, based on the principle that what is not used is lost. So people who claim that meat (or dairy products) do not agree with them are right. Their body is trying to tell them that if they eat these protein foods, they will not digest them anyway because they lack the HCl to do the job. Stress and lack of B vitamins also contribute to hydrochloric acid deficiency and many people lack it these days (some have none at all) yet they insist that, judging by their symptoms, they are already over-acid. TV and radio commercials joyfully perpetuate this myth in order to sell antacids. Yet research has shown that the symptoms of *too much acid* are *identical* with those of *too little acid*!

You can, of course, have a test to learn whether or not you lack HCl, but these tests are sometimes not too pleasant (like stomach pumping); or, if a simpler test is available, a doctor often is not convinced such a shortage exists, since the problem is little studied. Dr. Hugh Tuckey, a retired specialist in HCl deficiency and its correction, tells how you can test yourself.

In sum, he advocates the use of the supplement (from health stores) called HCl Betaine with Pepsin. It comes in tablet form, and Dr. Tuckey, after trying many different kinds of HCl, found this type most successful. He says to take one tablet immediately after a meal containing protein. If there is a burning sensation (extremely rare) drink a glass of water to wash it down. At the next meal, try ½ tablet. If the same symptoms occur, you may be the exception who does not need HCl (ulcer patients do not). On the other hand, if you feel no symptoms at all, this is good. I have had hundreds write me after reading this information in my book (9) that HCl has changed their indigestion and health for the better.

Alan H. Nittler, a nutritional M.D., starts his patients on a detoxifying diet to get rid of accumulated toxins in the body, eliminating protein for a short time only. Then he reinstates the patient on a medium amount of protein together with HCl if the patient needs it. He considers HCl one of the most important and most needed substances in this period of civilization. He believes that many people are forced into vegetarianism due to its lack.

What Kind of Protein?

There are two main types of vegetarians, those who eat no protein of any kind (known as vegans in Europe); and lacto-ovo-vegetarians. (*Lacto* means dairy or milk products; *ovo* means eggs.) Added to vegetables and fruits, these proteins make a well balanced diet, since they are complete proteins as well as contain B-12. Seventh-day Adventists are lacto-ovo-vegetarians; they have been tested many times, and been found to have an excellent health record.

Sometimes, even with the addition of some protein, a "hidden protein hunger" develops. I have seen this occur in some lacto-ovo-vegetarians who may compensate for a craving for larger amounts of protein with many carbohydrates, such as cakes, pies, cookies, and the like. This of course adds pounds and, unless the carbohydrates are natural ones, such as fruit, instead of man-made items, they are contraindicated for good health.

There is another problem in connection with dairy products. More and more people are finding they are allergic to milk and milk products (cheese, yogurt, etc., even if the milk is certified raw). This is because individuals as well as certain races lack an enzyme in their body known as lactase which is needed to assimilate lactose or milk sugar. Such people can sometimes, not always, tolerate the sour milks such as yogurt or kefir. If you notice allergic responses including mucus, you may have to give up the milk family. There is no commercial source of the enzyme lactase available. Some babies or adults are allergic to cow's milk but can take goat's milk or soy milk. Many adults who cannot take cow's milk can use cream successfully.

Soy protein is a complete protein and even contains some B-12, but although some people thrive on it, others do not. For these people it produces disturbing symptoms such as indigestion and gas, and is unacceptable. Soy protein is now used as a meat extender called TVP (textured vegetable protein). It is added to ground meat and displayed in supermarket meat counters. This problem has been thoroughly explained and documented by Beatrice Trum Hunter (10), who reminds us that even soy bakery products can disturb those who are allergic to it.

Dr. Bernard Jensen feels that we should eat a variety of proteins since certain amino acids, he believes, have specific actions for certain parts of the body. One may help the gall bladder, another the liver, and others serve different body organs. He adds, "Soybeans probably have most of the amino acids but not all. To rely on soybeans entirely would lead you toward a weakness in your health over a period of time due to this lack." (11)

Even flesh eaters have problems of choice. Not only are nonorganic meats questionable, but a diet of steaks or hamburger is less nutritious than liver and other organ meats, since organs are storage depots for vitamins and minerals.

Contaminated water can cause contaminated fish. There are more and more illnesses resulting from shell fish caught near the shore, and the safest fish, thus far, is that which comes from the deep sea. Freshwater fish should be judged by the condition of the water from which it was taken.

Chickens and eggs should be organic, if possible.

How to Set Up Your Own Diet

By now it has become clear that even if you are on a vegetarian diet, you need protein of some kind to keep your body intact and prevent that delayed reaction from catching up with you later. The type of protein is your own choice. Your preferences should be considered as well as any allergies.

How much protein should you include in your diet? Protein is measured in grams and the amount of protein usually recommended is 1 gram for each 2.2 pounds of body weight. A quick rule of thumb is to divide your weight in half and use one gram of protein daily for each remaining pound. For example, if you weigh 140 pounds, divide 140 into half, which would give you 70. That would mean on the average that 70 grams of protein are a good average daily amount for you. If you are a hard physical or mental worker, or have been ill, or are pregnant, you might need more, but the half-of-your-weight amount is probably a good overall standard.

Richard Talbot, the only vegetarian-minded person I have ever known who remained healthy and energetic, includes some fish or dairy product in his diet and computes his protein supply daily. If his supply is short, he makes it up before going to bed. He has written a helpful little booklet called *How to Count Your Grams of Protein*. This is available by request at health stores. I will sum up Richard Talbot's findings here:

Concerning Recommended Amount of Protein

"The heart alone needs 50 grams of the finest protein available every twenty-four hours."

"All human beings after the age of twelve require approximately 75 grams of high-grade protein daily. Under age twelve, half that amount is sufficient."

"Those who refuse to listen to scientists and insist that they can derive all the protein their bodies need from seeds, nuts or beans ... are the dreamy visionaries ... We have watched them over the years and one by one they have ended up with disastrous consequences." The time for delayed reaction differs; the results are always similar.

Concerning Protein Rating in Order of Importance

1. Eggs (forget about cholesterol, its "danger" is a myth for eggs) (12)
2. Milk and cheese
3. Flesh (meat, fish and poultry)

"Flesh food eaten once a day is enough and should be eaten with the evening meal, together with cooked vegetables and a raw salad," Mr. Talbot says. He also suggests taking 25 grams of protein at each meal to get your total 75 grams daily.

If you are trying to get 25 grams per meal, and run short, you could round out with a few protein tablets, *providing* they are first class protein. These protein supplements usually come in powder form, too. Read your labels to determine from which source they are derived: eggs, milk, soy or whatever. Although I am not a vege-

How to Compute Your Own Diet (13)

Sources of Complete Proteins plus B-12	Amounts	Grams of Protein
Soybean flour (low fat)	1 cup	60
Wheat germ	½ cup	24
Brewer's yeast, powdered (includes B-12 if so labeled)	½ cup	50
Egg	1	6
Milk, whole, skim, buttermilk	1 quart	32-35
Cottage cheese	½ cup	20
American or Swiss cheese	2 slices	10-12
Soybeans, cooked	½ cup	20
Meat, fish, fowl	¼ lb.	15-22

(approximately 1 serving)

tarian, I use the Malabar tablets and powder mentioned in "Body Regeneration." Remember, these are pure, unadulterated glandular proteins without additives, sugar, fillers or chemicals. Two tablets equal one gram, a convenience if you need a small addition to complete your protein total. Two tablespoons of the powder equal 27 grams. The flavor is not exactly palatable because it is the real thing, but combined with brewer's yeast in juice it becomes a powerhouse. Brewer's yeast alone is a terrific food, an energy builder deluxe. It not only is a complete protein containing all of the essential amino acids, but also contains all B vitamins (including B-12, if so bred). A tablespoon at a time taken in juice or water between meals produces an energy pickup far more rewarding and longer lasting than coffee.

A new protein powder has recently arrived on the market: Super 15. It is a whole food, a complete protein with B-12, as the following analysis shows:

alfalfa
wheat germ
soy amino acids, pre-digested, complete protein
rice polish

food yeast with B-12
sea kelp
lecithin
soy meal
alfalfa seed
chia seed
pumpkin seed
sesame seed
sunflower seed
enzymes

It has a pleasant flavor and is a complete food containing vitamins and minerals as well as protein. You could actually live on it. One heaping tablespoon equals 17.5 grams of protein or 5.7 grams of carbohydrate, or 80 calories.

Protein is extremely important as you have seen. But it is not the whole story. Vitamins, minerals, enzymes (either digestive or those from fresh fruits and vegetables to assist many body functions) plus oils are necessary for good health, too. For those people on a high protein diet, added calcium may be needed. This is because protein is high in phosphorus and there should be a balance of calcium-phosphorus in the body at a ratio of 2½ : 1. Otherwise if there is more phosphorus than calcium, the calcium shortage may become manifest as nervousness, leg cramps, etc. which disappear when calcium is added. Vitamin B-6 is also recommended for high protein diets, to keep the body in balance.

There has been an observation (so far unverified to my knowledge) that diets high in minerals require less protein. This may explain why the Hunzas, who eat little protein, are so well; their water is thick with minerals from glacial silt. It may also explain why Orientals are healthy on little protein. They use much mineral-rich seaweed.

You will find many arguments against animal protein

by so called "experts" as well as by vegetarians themselves. A little discretion is called for here. For example, one report insists that mushrooms contain as much protein as meat. Actually there are about 10 grams (average) of protein in one pound of mushrooms (14) as compared with 15 to 22 grams in one-fourth pound of meat. There is also the statement that mushrooms contain B-12. Since B-12 is measured in micrograms, one would have to eat a lot of mushrooms to get the daily requirement. One can eat only so many mushrooms, and at the present price of roughly $1.00 per pound, they are not a bargain.

Other recent reports state that the amount of protein suggested: one gram for each 2.2 pounds of body weight, is out of date and much less is now needed. I challenge this statement. The amount of protein needed is based upon the individual. Hard physical workers need far more than sedentary workers. Pregnant women need far more than non-pregnant women. And in these days of great stress and strain on bodies and glands, more, not less, may be necessary to keep up one's resistance.

By the same token of individual difference, however, the type of protein may vary. One person may find that he can assimilate fowl or fish better than beef or lamb. If so, he must abide by the needs of his own body.

The problem is not to go overboard. One nutrition researcher in good standing tells of the tragic case of a young boy, who, due to the restrictions of a religious sect ate only raw food, interspersed with weekly fasts, for many months. He had one nervous breakdown, was on the verge of another, and was skin and bones as well as mentally confused and subject to abnormal fits of anger (15).

A reader wrote me recently as follows:

"I am a vegetarian and believe I have not been getting enough protein, living mostly on fruit. I have become very weak. The doctor recently found an interior growth which he said was due to lack of hormones. I feel sure it is due to the fact that I am 'falling apart' due to lack of protein. I hope this information will help others who insist on becoming vegetarian."

To complete this answer to your letter, E. B., I do hope this information helps your Zen groups. Richard Talbot states, "The secret of having successful bodies is to give them not what *we* desire, but what *they* require! If we do, they will rarely malfunction."

I believe that with the above scientific information plus pencil and paper, any person can work out a vegetarian diet for his particular needs and follow it successfully for life.

Sincerely,
Linda Clark

References

1. Christopher Bird and Peter Tompkins. *The Secret Life of Plants*. New York, N.Y.: Avon Books, 1974.

2. Linda Clark. *Secrets of Health and Beauty*. New York, N.Y.: Pyramid Publications, 1970.

3. Dr. Bernard Jensen. *World Keys to Health and Longevity*. Escondido, Cal.: Omni Publishers, 1975.

4. Adelle Davis. *Let's Eat Right to Keep Fit*. New York, N.Y.: New American Library, 1970.

5. *American Journal of Orthodontics and Oral Surgery*. August 1946.

6. Frances Moore Lappé. *Diet for a Small Planet*. Rev. ed. New York, N.Y.: Ballantine Books, 1975.

7. *Organic Gardening*. June 1975.

8 *The New York Times.* 21 March 1975

9. *Secrets of Health and Beauty.*

10. *Consumer's Research Magazine.* February 1974.

11. *World Keys to Health and Longevity.*

12. Linda Clark. *Know Your Nutrition.* New Canaan, Conn Keats Publishing, 1973.

13 *Let's Eat Right to Keep Fit.*

14. United States Department of Agriculture Handbook No. 8: *Composition of Foods.*

15. Mary Jane Hungerford. "Common Behavior Patterns." *Journal of Applied Nutrition.* Vol. 27, no. 4. Winter 1975.

Container Gardening

ONE SPRING, for the first time in years I found myself without an organic garden. Circumstances had forced me to sell my home and the surrounding acreage, and I had moved temporarily into a small rented house with almost no yard.

Discussing my plight with a friend, he made what I thought an absurd suggestion, considering I was in temporary quarters and had only about a seven-foot strip of land around the house. "Just plant another garden," he said.

He explained he was talking about "container gardening" and chided me for my skepticism. He said he had turned to this method of gardening when he discovered the soil on his land was too hard and that getting it in shape would have been an extremely expensive proposition.

In a half-hearted way, I decided to give it a try. I collected every type of container I could find—large clay pots, as many five-gallon cans as a nursery could spare, wooden boxes of every description, including old flats which had formerly held seedlings from a nursery. I discovered a child's sandbox in the yard and purchased a few half-barrels from a winery.

To the garden soil, I added some dried manure, a little sand and some mushroom compost obtained from a nearby mushroom farm. In each container I planted a few seeds of a single species—yellow summer squash in one, zucchini in another, cucumbers in two more, climbing Kentucky Wonder green beans in another and a tomato plant in still another. In the flats I planted lettuce, spinach, radishes, and onion sets. In the child's sandbox I planted chard as well as pepper and eggplants.

I listlessly watered the containers, now planted, still dreaming about my large organic garden. I had to admit, though, that it had been hard work outwitting gophers and moles in my old garden. There is nothing more discouraging than to go to bed at night with the garden full of luxurious squash, cucumber and thriving potato plants, and wake up in the morning to find many destroyed from beneath the surface, the plants lying flat and inert on the ground. Poison is out because of pets. Even trapping has its drawbacks; a pet cat or dog can be injured by digging at the scent of the pesky rodents. And without pesticides, which I refuse to use, I was also forced to admit that many treasured plants had been attacked and destroyed by snails, earwigs, raccoons, rabbits and deer. As soon as we found a fence or other control for one, another would take over.

Now as I watered my little containers, there was no sign of predators. I began to cheer up.

In due time, the seeds came up and grew into plants. Lettuce, radishes and spinach were first available as food. Later came a riotous array of everything else, which bore prolifically. While I did not have a great surplus to share with neighbors, it was all I could do to keep up with eating the produce myself. I tallied up seventy-five cucumbers from two containers—far more than from many more vines in my other garden. I had all the spinach, beans, summer squash, and later, peppers, eggplants, onions and tomatoes I could use.

Small winter squash also thrived. The prize tomato plant produced late and huge tomatoes in spite of being broken off by a dog jumping on it from over a fence. It rallied and began all over again. As I am writing this in late October, I have just brought it in as a house plant

174

(together with a pepper plant) and it is even more luxurious than it was. At the moment, it contains eighteen tomatoes in various sizes, some of them weighing up to a pound.

There are many advantages of container gardening. Containers are portable and can be moved from one part of the property to another (or from one house to another). They can be moved into or out of the sun as the seasons change. By slipping one or more large plastic garbage bags over them, they can become miniature greenhouses to protect them from frost and carry some plants over the winter until spring planting time.

Although crops such as corn undeniably need more space, an unbelievable variety of edibles can be raised, including potatoes, a small orchard and berries. In *The Book of Survival*, Edmond Bordeaux Szekely states that a dozen containers of dwarf varieties of fruit trees can ensure an excellent supply of fruit and that sixteen square yards of space can provide one person with an abundant annual supply of vegetables. Furthermore, foods not available elsewhere can be raised, and there is a definite financial as well as health benefit. Work, weeds and cultivation are reduced to a minimum.

The easiest method of cultivation and enrichment of the soil for container gardening can be done with the help of earthworms. These little wrigglers (a special variety used for this purpose may be available in your own area or advertised in organic gardening magazines; just plain earthworms aren't as successful) can be great helpers. They aerate the soil, digest it, make it friable and rich. They are also the best kind of garbage disposal known.

Although I have a regular garbage disposal in the sink, I never use it. Instead, the earthworms do the job for me. In a large, outdoor, wooden box (a barrel will do) you can put several inches of soil on the bottom, add

500 to 1,000 earthworms, and cover again with soil. Adding some dry, old rotted manure (available at nurseries, supermarkets and garden shops) helps. Fresh manure becomes too hot and burns. Several times a week I add my table scraps. With a trowel, I make an indentation in the soil, bury the scraps and cover again with the soil. Usually, when I am ready to add more scraps, the previous addition has disappeared and the worms have proliferated.

Given food and water, without which they will die, they multiply faster than rabbits. Earthworms like cornmeal, coffee grounds, fat drippings, crushed eggshells, all peelings and any other scraps you can spare. I add more soil as needed, sometimes topping the pile with leaves and weeds as a mulch to preserve the moisture. In other words, I return everything (except citrus rinds, which break down too slowly) to the soil and the earthworms take it from there. There should be no odor and no flies. The box should also be placed in shade or semi-shade so the worms will not get too hot and dry during hot weather.

Those who live in colder climates can use this "garbage disposal, soil-enrichment method" on a year-round basis in their basements. When I lived on the East Coast, I got seven flats, added soil, a few earthworms, and labeled each flat with the name of the day of the week. I placed the flats on the basement floor. On Monday, I buried Monday's table scraps in the Monday box. On Tuesday, I repeated the process. By the time I got around to Monday again, there were no scraps left; only rich soil and a few more earthworms. There was absolutely no odor. The basement smelled as fresh as a greenhouse. In the spring, I transferred the surplus worms to the outdoor garden.

In my container garden, I planted a few scraggly tomato plants in the compost box. Because of the shade, there were fewer tomatoes but the stalks were so vigorous they resembled small trees, confirmation of the richness of the soil provided by the earthworms. I added some of this same soil, plus earthworms, to all containers.

Because of the earthworms, I do not bother to have my soil tested for acidity or alkalinity. According to Mr. Szekely, the humus produced by the worms can correct over-acidity or over-alkalinity. In his book, he suggests this simple method of testing: Mix up a little of your garden soil with a small amount of water, shake and let settle. From the drug store buy some strips of litmus paper, which turns red if exposed to acidity, or blue when alkaline, or remains grey if the mixture is neutral. If you find over-acidity, or over-alkalinity, merely add some more worm-humus for correction.

There are a few other pointers to keep in mind when planting your containers. The containers should have drainage holes in the bottom. Small-gauge screen netting should be placed over the holes to prevent earthworms from escaping. For plants with shallow roots, six or seven inches of soil are sufficient, whereas eight to twelve inches are needed for deeper root systems. Tomatoes are said to need several feet to sink their roots, but mine thrived on twelve inches of soil and produced many huge, delicious fruit.

It is also necessary to water containers daily in hot weather, for the sake of both the plants and the earthworms. You can test the moisture by sticking your finger an inch or so down into the soil. Once a week I fertilized with liquid fish emulsion, diluting it according to directions on the label. Except for picking the produce, that was all the work required.

What can you raise in containers? In my own garden, in addition to the vegetables already mentioned, I grew every variety of herb, including comfrey and several kinds of mint.

My friend who got me interested in container gardening has raised the following edibles in containers:

Vegetables

asparagus
pole beans
artichokes (Jerusalem and American)
celery (it grew head high)
lettuce
radishes
carrots
beets
chard
onions
tomatoes
peppers
eggplant
cabbage
melons
sunflowers for seed
potatoes (in wine barrels, with straw mulch)

Fruits
(all trees are dwarf)

apples (several varieties)
peaches
pears
persimmons
apricots
cherries
plums
oranges
lemons
limes

178

grapefruit
tangerines
loquats
pomegranates
figs

Berries

strawberries
blueberries
raspberries
blackberries
boysenberries
grapes (six varieties)

Flower-lovers can be equally successful. Another container gardener raises seventy-five varieties of flowers on the deck of his San Francisco apartment, despite the fog and wind. He hand mixes inland sand, redwood chips, topsoil or potting mix, and Irish moss, all obtained from a garden shop. He, too, feeds his plants liquid fish emulsion. Another friend in my area plants bulbs in many pots, bringing them out from hiding and massing them for dramatic effect, replacing them with other later-blooming varieties as the old ones die down.

I now have acquired more land, with space for a larger garden. But because of the water shortage in California where I live, as well as the cement-like hardness of the soil in the summertime, a peculiarity of this state, I have never returned to full-scale gardening in the ground.

I brought with me all the containers collected in my temporary quarters and have had new ones built, with small-mesh wire screen on the bottom of large, deep flats, to protect against gophers and moles. Actually, except for large plants such as corn, summer squash and bush beans, the plants raised in my containers produced more abundant crops than similar species raised in the ground. The reason. It is easier to control not only pests, but watering and fertilizing.

What started as an apparent disaster turned out to be a blessing in disguise. I now plan always to practice this method of "armchair gardening."